YOUR GUIDE TO HYPNOBIRTHING

The Rose Method

Rose Byrne

Available in paperback, ebook and audiobook

For Amanda,

Wishing you a calm, empowered birth.

Rose,

xx

Copyright © 2024 Rose Byrne

All rights reserved

The knowledge, information and experiences portrayed in this book are an amalgamation of what I have taught & learnt from the many couples I have worked with, and that which I read, researched and used during my own pregnancy, labour and birth. Testimonials and birth stories have been shared with permission.

No part of this book may be reproduced, or stored in a retrieval system, or transmitted in any form or by any means, electronic, mechanical, photocopying, recording, or otherwise, without express written permission of the publisher.

ISBN-13 (paperback): 9798883895660
ASIN (ebook): B0CW1PWC2J

Cover design by: Art Painter (photo by Rose Byrne)
Printed by Kindle Direct Publishing
Library of Congress Control Number: 2018675309

Cover Image

The unfiltered, unedited photograph on the front of this book was captured by the author, in November 2023, and is of Caylee and Omar enjoying a relaxation exercise during one of their Rose Method Hypnobirthing classes. Shared with permission.

*Dedicated to Orla without whom this book wouldn't have happened. Keep shining bright and never let anyone dull your sparkle!
Love always, from Mum xx*

CONTENTS

Title Page
Copyright
Dedication
Acknowledgements & Gratitude   6
    11
HOUR ONE   18
HOUR TWO   42
HOUR THREE   62
HOUR FOUR   70
HOUR FIVE   76
HOUR SIX   80
HOUR SEVEN   90
HOUR EIGHT   102
HOUR NINE   114
HOUR 10   124
HOUR 11   136
HOUR 12   154
About The Author   198

What's Covered In Each Chapter?

Acknowledgements & Gratitude - Words of appreciation for those who encouraged, inspired & believed in me

Conception - This is the introduction

Hour One - The history & philosophy of hypnobirthing

Hour Two - The uterus

Hour Three - You can have a calm birth. Words of Conscious Reaffirmation

Hour Four - Anchors (part 1)

Hour Five - Anchors (part 2)

Hour Six - Surge breathing

Hour Seven - The umbilical cord, the placenta, skin-to-skin & Vitamin K

Hour Eight - Estimated due dates & avoiding unnecessary medical induction

Hour Nine - Your body is working for you & perineal massage

Hour 10 - Labour day, the purple line & making your way to the birth centre

Hour 11 - Birth breathing

Hour 12 - How do you feel about labour & birth now & how do you think it will be? Parents' Promise & Ways to Practise & Prepare for Your Hypnobirth

Birth Stories & Testimonials for The Rose Method

Let others know what you thought of the book

Rose's online links

About the author

ACKNOWLEDGEMENTS & GRATITUDE

I'm grateful to each and every one of the following, amazing people who have played a part in my journey towards birthing this book. These names are in no particular order.

All of my clients – I'm honoured to have been a special part of the birth preparation journey for lots of wonderful couples. Many of them encouraged me to write my own method and accompanying book before I had seriously considered it myself and they became my inspiration as I could see how I was helping them have calm, positive births. Thank you to those who read the draft version of this book as part of their hypnobirthing course before the book was finished. I especially want to mention Lucy and Eddo who said, before I even started writing this book, that I definitely have what it takes to create my own method and that if I stop teaching hypnobirthing, that it would be like if Madonna stopped writing music – there would still be music but no Madonna. I'll take that – being thought of as the Madonna of Hypnobirthing!

Orla – for being the reason it all happened 16 years ago. I hope I'm raising you to know that you can be whoever you want to be as you find your own path in life. Shine bright and never let anyone dull your sparkle

My dad – For always being there, for raising me to have a good work ethic and for paying towards my place on Suzy Ashworth's Mykonos retreat during my fiftieth year. That trip was such a catalyst.

Pete – For being my rock during pregnancy, labour and birth and for doing the hypnobirthing with me despite initially describing a hypnobirthing practitioner as 'another hippy after my money'. You were then totally blown away by how calm and quiet I was once the time came to use what Katharine had taught me. I even recall a few weeks later, how you told your sister that she should do hypnobirthing if she has any more children.

Kathy – For believing in me and for telling me for years that I should write my own method. Also, for being the best friend I could ask for and the best godmother to Orla.

My late mum – As I go through this journey of life, I carry with me all the wisdom and unconditional love that my mum gave me. I remember Mum being very proud of my work as a hypnobirthing teacher and she enjoyed reading my clients' birth stories and reviews. I don't believe in coincidences – I believe that everything happens for a reason. On the one-year anniversary of Mum's death, I received a call from a lady wanting to do hypnobirthing with me. I wasn't really answering calls that day as I was spending time with my dad and my daughter, remembering Mum. But something made me take that call. The lady on the phone was quite far along in her pregnancy and we agreed it would be good to get started with one-to-one sessions soon and that those could take place in the comfort of her own home. When she told me her address, it sent shivers up my spine and left me speechless. She lived in the house that my mum had also lived in from the day she was born until she was 23 years old. I taught hypnobirthing in my mum's childhood home and that phone call on the anniversary of her death felt like a message somehow.

Katharine Graves – For being a hypnobirthing teacher when I was pregnant when there was nobody local to me and for coming to my home. I will always remember that lovely day sitting in my garden with you and learning how to release my fears and to believe in myself and in my ability to experience a calm labour and birth. Thank you so much.

The late Marie Mongan (1933-2019) - founder of The Mongan Method and grandmother of Hypnobirthing – Such a legend who has left a legacy, having made birth better for thousands of women worldwide! When I was pregnant myself in 2007, I was taught The Mongan Method by Katharine Graves. I then went on to train as a Mongan Method practitioner in 2010 and was thrilled when, upon receiving my theory work back in the post from New Hampshire, I saw that Marie had marked it herself. I felt so proud and will always treasure that as well as my Hypnobirthing Institute certificate, also signed by Marie. My one regret is that I never got to meet Marie in-person.

Alan Davidson – my hypnotherapy lecturer from May 2009

until April 2010. My birth experience in 2007 was so very calm and life changing, and I wanted to find out how that had been possible when just weeks before, I was petrified of the prospect of giving birth. I am very grateful to you for helping me understand the role which the conscious and subconscious areas of my mind played in my ability to labour and birth without fear. Thank you for being such a fabulous teacher and making your hypnotherapy and counselling diploma course so interesting.

Leila – For being my hypnobirthing colleague and an amazing, supportive friend over the last decade.

Lucinda – I am so grateful to Lucinda for her patience with me and believing that I could and would do this. I am so happy that Lucinda asked to train under me as a hypnobirthing practitioner sharing The Rose Method. Lucinda also recommended my first ever client to me back in 2010.

Tamara Cianfini – I have on DVD some of the births Tamara attended as a doula and these have enabled all of my clients to see hypnobirthing successfully put into practice. This definitely helped them go on to have positive birth experiences themselves. Thanks to Tamara for also providing comfort and advice when I phoned her after receiving some upsetting news just before teaching a hypnobirthing class. I will always remember and feel grateful to you.

Elena Tonetti-Vladimirova – When I was pregnant, my own hypnobirthing practitioner showed me some births on the Birth into Being DVD. This definitely helped me to see birth more positively. I later invested in my own copy – it's truly a wonderful film and I especially loved learning about the Black Sea Birth Camps.

The late Edith Cotterill (my great aunt & author of Nurse on Call) – I think a little of Auntie Bob's talent and passion for writing has found its way into my DNA and for this I am truly grateful.

Neil - When our paths first crossed, I'd been putting off getting this book finished and published. '*We* need to get that book out there!' you told me a few weeks after we met. No one else had said it like that to me before. I just got on with it after that. Thank you! x

Suzy Ashworth – Wow, Suzy! Thank you for Message Mastery, The Wealth Frequency Playbook, all the Thrive Thursdays but most of all for that retreat in Mykonos – Boom! Now THAT was life changing and such a catalyst for me! Faith + Action really does equal Miracles!

The Mykonos Magic ladies - They say we become like the people we surround ourselves with and I have been fortunate to stay in-touch with you all. Every one of you has inspired me so much since that life-changing retreat in 2022.

Florence Andrews – For speaking in a way that meant I finally understood what it would take to become the version of myself I needed to be to finally get this book and my method out there. Elevate was incredible!

Becky – For being a wonderful friend since we were 16 when we met over a box of chocolates at college, for giving sound advice and for being almost as excited as I was about publishing this book.

Scott Buckley – for composing the beautiful music 'Adrift Amongst Infinite Stars' which I found on chosic.com and which plays in the background on all the MP3s that accompany The Rose Method.

Kevin Long (aka The Kindle King) – for his time and inspiring words of wisdom as a fantastic publisher. I highly recommend Kevin to any of you who want to get your book out there.

CONCEPTION.

Why did I write this book?

This book has primarily been written to accompany The Rose Method antenatal hypnobirthing course. You have probably been given this copy by your hypnobirthing practitioner. If however, you have started to read this and are pregnant but have not yet booked your classes, please get in-touch by emailing me at rose@bournecalm.com so that I can help you find a suitable hypnobirthing practitioner for you to discuss your options with.

What is Hypnobirthing?

The knowledge, information and experience I have shared in this book comes from within me - what I learnt first-hand as a mum to be, things I read and researched, techniques I used myself during pregnancy, labour and birth in 2007, and it's also an amalgamation of what I have taught (and learnt) from the many couples I have worked with since 2010 as East Dorset's longest-running, award-winning hypnobirthing practitioner, trained and experienced in The Mongan, Wise Hippo and KG methods of this life-changing, calming and empowering way to approach and prepare yourself for birth.

I haven't always been into hypnotherapy, hypnobirthing and all things calm birth. When I carried my B.B (Baby Byrne), the tiny human that was growing inside of me, I felt a love and a connection I didn't even know could exist for another person. I used to dance to the David Bowie cover of 'Wild is The Wind' with my hands on my (at that time) still small belly. I felt so vulnerable in those early, fragile months of pregnancy. And BB grew and grew. I was in awe of what my body was doing, even though I didn't understand as much about it then as I do now.

'I hear the sound of mandolins
Oh, kiss me
With your kiss my life begins
You're spring to me, all things to me
Don't you know you're life itself?
Like the leaf clings to the tree,
Oh my darling, cling to me
For we're like creatures of the wind
And wild is the wind
Wild is the wind'

– Wild is The Wind cover by David Bowie (lyrics originally written by Dimitri Tiomkin and Ned Washington).

My Hypnobirthing journey started when, in 2007, at 26 weeks pregnant, my baby-bump had just started showing and I had told the HR department where I worked at the time, that I was having a baby. A few of the ladies at work had young children already. My colleague Debbie had attended an NCT course and mentioned that one of the women on that course hadn't had, or needed for that matter, any pain relief during labour and birth. Debbie had said that, as far as she was aware, the only thing this woman had done differently was to have hypnotherapy during her pregnancy. So, on the back of that, I did go for some hypnotherapy sessions around 28 weeks. But at that point I was still totally unaware that hypnobirthing existed.

As a pregnant woman, very frightened of giving birth, it was only when I read Callie's birth story on a pregnancy forum (this was just before Facebook or any other social media platforms were in the common domain) that I first saw the word hypnobirthing mentioned anywhere by anyone. From what Callie was saying, her labour and birth was not without complication, but it was without panic. It read as though Callie had been in a sleep-like state through much of her labour whilst, at the same time, being very much aware and in control of everything that her body was doing. Hers was the most inspiring birth story I had ever come across. There it was! I had discovered the existence of the word 'hypnobirthing'. At 38 weeks pregnant, after reading the single most positive, inspiring account of birth I had come across in my life until that point, I knew this was something else – it was different from the hypnotherapy sessions I had been to on the back of my colleague's recommendation – Hypnobirthing was more than hypnotherapy. I knew with complete certainty that I would commit myself to finding someone to show me how I could experience labour in that way; like Callie had. To birth in a way without fear, pain and screaming.

And there was no one, it seemed. No one to show me the hypnobirthing way Callie had described - no one who understood what I was looking for - not here or nearby.

A Google search for hypnobirthing brought nothing up in the Bournemouth or surrounding areas and I settled for sending emails to several local hypnotherapists. I asked them if they were familiar with hypnobirthing, and could they teach it to me? It was a Saturday evening so I closed the laptop and went to sit in the lounge in the hope that I would receive answers back from my enquiries on Monday morning. And then you phoned me - Katharine Graves - you lived quite far away but you immediately reassured me, and a couple of days later, you sent me a book called Hypnobirthing by Marie Mongan and some relaxation tracks on a cd to play when I was about to go to sleep each night. I was cutting it a bit fine, you said, but yes, you would be able to teach me the birth preparation method I'd just read about in Callie's birth story. And that moment was my gateway to Hypnobirthing. Katharine Graves would be my practitioner.

I felt a little bit excited and very relieved then because I started to see that there could be another way for me.

I started reading Hypnobirthing by Marie Mongan on the day I received my copy from Katharine. Near the start of the book, Marie included some accounts written by British doctor, Grantly

Dick-Read about his experiences attending home and hospital births. One line sent shivers up my spine the first time I read it and it still gives me goose bumps now – so powerful were those words for me there and then, as they are the words that spell out the reason why I, like so many others, was petrified about the prospect of giving birth and yet other women are very relaxed about it. Here is the excerpt from the book including that poignant line. I wonder if you will feel goose bumps after reading it too:

"Dr. Dick-Read first became sensitive to the true nature of labour and birth in a humble, poverty-ridden setting in London in 1913. As a young intern in London's Whitechapel district in the heart of the East End slums, he was called to attend a woman in labour. After travelling on his bicycle through mud and rain, he arrived at about three in the morning at a low hovel near some railroad arches. He found his way to a small apartment where he discovered his patient in a dim room, soaked from the rain pouring in from the leaky roof. She was covered only with sacks and an old black skirt. He asked permission to put the mask over her face and administer chloroform. Her emphatic refusal was a first for Dick-Read. He returned the chloroform and mask to his bag, stood back and watched as she, with little more than gentle breathing, birthed her baby. The baby was born with little fuss or noise from the mother. As he prepared to leave, Dick-Read asked why she had refused the relief from pain.

She gave him an answer that he was never to forget.

'It didn't hurt. It wasn't supposed to, was it, Doctor?'"

I remember reading that line and then reading it again. The message was a simple one, but it was immediately very meaningful for me. No one had told the Whitechapel woman that labour and birth were painful. I started to wonder if it was possible that I only feared labour and birth as much as I'd been conditioned to. Had I ever been told anything positive about the birth process? Was it too late? I would never be able to 'unhear' those bad things, would I? It wasn't possible to reverse being told something, surely. Well, the amazing news is that despite negative information being seven times more memorable by the brain than positive information, it is definitely possible to reprogramme our minds so that we can learn, believe and retain new information on a topic we already hold previously stored information about. As you read through this book and work through your course, you are going to learn how you can do exactly that.

Recently, I posted a letter of appreciation to Katharine Graves on LinkedIn. Here is an excerpt:

'And then I met you, Katharine, and you taught me so much that day when you came to my home.
And yet I still couldn't believe that I would be 'as good' as the women in those calm birthing videos you showed me.
And do you remember what you said to me?
You simply said, 'But why wouldn't you be? You are like them. And how do you know that those women didn't do hypnobirthing because when they were pregnant, they felt exactly the same fear as you do now?'
Thank you.'

'When you change the way you view birth, the way you birth will change.' – Marie Mongan (1933-2019) - founder of Hypnobirthing.

I breathe slowly whilst visualising through each of my powerful surges.

HOUR ONE

Upon meeting your Rose Method Hypnobirthing practitioner and introducing yourselves, you'll have been asked to work either by yourself or together with your partner on an exercise. You will have then written down some things about how you were feeling about labour and birth at that point and your thoughts on how you expect your birth experience to be before having done any hypnobirthing. I think it's especially good to do this as a couple. Partners are going through a big change in their life too and focusing on how you both feel and being open with each other about this is a way to bring you closer. Some couples do this within their relationship anyway. It's certainly a beneficial exercise because most of the time the focus is on how the person* carrying and birthing the baby is doing with far less regard for the other parent*.

*Since teaching hypnobirthing to same-sex couples and non-binaries, I no longer assume that each couple comprises of an expectant mum and her male partner, hence why I use the terms 'the person carrying and birthing the baby' and 'the other parent'. I have also taught women who have chosen a donor to conceive or who find themselves single for another reason. In these cases, I do recommend that your birth partner (friend, sister, mum, doula) attend classes together with you if possible. However, my course has been attended without partners many times and that works too. Lisa has done hypnobirthing with me three times and her husband was her rock during each of their birth experiences. The two of them enjoyed what they called hypnobirthing date nights once a week during which Lisa briefed her husband on what we had covered at that week's class and they practised techniques at home together at least once a week too.

Here are some of the things expectant parents have written during that very first exercise during their course:

Painful

Apprehensive

Nervous

Scared

So many different choices – scared to choose the wrong one

I hope the baby will be healthy and ok

I don't want to be induced

Having such a long weary labour

Excited

Adrenaline

I hope I can do it naturally but the thought scares me

I can't wait to meet my baby

Unpredictable

Messy

Unprepared

Scary

Stressful

Worried

Worried because it was so difficult last time – I am doing this because I need it to be different this time

It will be hard seeing my partner in pain

I am going to have to get everything ready beforehand

I don't want to go to hospital

If I could avoid the giving birth part, I would

I don't want a Caesarean

A bit panicky in case I lose control because I think that could make it worse

I don't think my partner knows / has a clue what is actually going to happen which stresses me out

It will be a big drain on my body

Excited to learn

Nervous about complications

I am feeling apprehensive about giving birth

I am not good with pain

Trying to process the thought of what is going to happen is making me feel very nervous and scared

I don't feel mentally ready

I am feeling excited about becoming a parent

I am a little worried about my wife giving birth

Relaxed

Confident

Anxious about the size of the baby

Slightly anxious over the pain

Concerned in case I won't give birth naturally

I'm frightened that I can't do it

I believe there will be some pain but I am confident it can be manageable

What if my preference of birth place isn't suitable?

Confident but aware that things might not go to plan

A bit scared but confident

Hoping it will be less traumatic this time

Happy to be having our second child

Worried about contractions

That's just a selection. At the end of the course, your practitioner will return your sheet to you and ask you the same two questions. You'll have the opportunity to write your answers on the back of the sheet and will then be able to compare each set of answers after completing the exercise for the second time. This demonstrates how transformative the course truly is. At the back of the book, I have shared some examples of parents' 'after' feelings and thoughts.

I am the expert of my body.

How this book will benefit you throughout your hypnobirthing course
and on the lead up to your baby's birth.

The sections of this book are divided into 'hours' instead of chapters. I decided on this format so that if you want to read some of the book between your hypnobirthing sessions, the section you read will be relevant to and reaffirm what was covered in your most recent class. When we are learning new information, the average brain can concentrate for about 20 minutes before naturally wanting to switch off and process briefly, but everyone is different, and each person will find some information more interesting and worthy of remembering than other information. Reading the book can help fill in any focus attention-span gaps.

When I was writing this book, I read about an idea called 'the curse of knowledge' coined by the psychologist and linguist Steven Pinker. He says that the more of an expert you are in something, the more likely it is that you will associate with other people who are experts in that area. When that happens, it becomes harder to bridge the gap to what non-experts can understand. It's all too easy to start assuming too much knowledge on behalf of other people. I have been mindful not to use too much 'birthy' terminology and to make this book easy to read. If anything doesn't make sense, please either let your practitioner or me know.

Your classes will likely be three hours long. However, the course has been written in a such a way that it can be split up into anything from 12 x one-hour sessions or 2 x six-hour sessions (ie a weekend course from 10am until 4pm on both the Saturday and the Sunday). After each class, I'd recommend reading the hours associated with what was covered during that class.

The History and Philosophy of Hypnobirthing

Unfortunately, most people in the western world today, believe they're lucky if they don't need medical assistance, whereas the truth is that you're highly unlikely to need it.

Birth is a natural event that occasionally requires medical assistance. Sadly, it is seen by most as a medical event that occasionally happens naturally.

Statistics tell us that 31% / 28% / 34.5% of babies born in England / Wales / Scotland respectively in 2019 / 2020 were caesarean section births.

Here are the birth statistics for October 2023 at Epsom and St Helier University Hospitals:

352 babies born

3 home births (0.85%)

Birth Centre 12.9%

Labour Ward 85.4%

Babies born in water 5.68%

Labours induced 39.8%

Caesarean births 37.4% (that's more than twice the safe level of surgical birth according to the World Health Organisation)

10.6% Ventouse / forceps extraction

Over in the US, the caesarean rate was 32.1% in 2021.

I refuse to believe that one third of women are unable to birth vaginally. Remember, the human body only knows one way for a baby to be born. Our bodies and our babies are unaware of the existence of surgical birth.

However, there are places even in developed countries of the world where the statistics tell a very different story. The caesarean rate at The Farm's midwifery clinic in Summertown, Tennessee is less than 2%. This surely highlights the stark differences in birth centre practices, and I believe it demonstrates that a lot of hospital staff are working in fear, a fear which is often transferred to, and affects the experience for, the labouring mum, her partner and her baby – this certainly seems to be the case when a woman is under consultant-led care during her pregnancy. Consultants only get involved when there is a complication, meaning that they have only seen complicated births and this will understandably impact their view of birth.

The following is taken from www.thefarmmidwives.org:

'In 1970, over 200 visionaries left San Francisco on a quest for a new way of life that would establish a stronger connection to the values of humanity. A powerful element in this voyage of discovery was the belief that the sanctity of birth should be returned to the family. Birth was regarded as a natural and fulfilling experience that empowered women and bonded the family together.

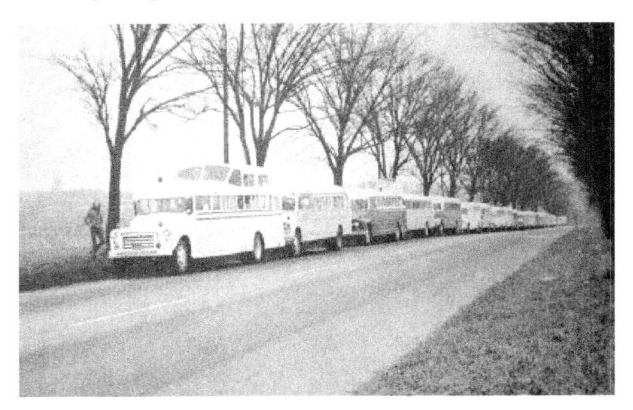

Photo courtesy of www.thefarmmidwives.org

The first births took place in school buses parked at various stops as the group travelled across the country. In all 11 babies were born on the road. Right away it became apparent that those attending the mother and baby carried a responsibility that was not to be taken lightly, and that knowledge and training were necessary to manage common complications of birth.

The Caravan came to a stop on 1750 acres in Middle Tennessee, to become The Farm Community. Spiritual seekers and cultural revolutionaries came from all across the world, growing from the original 200 to over 1200 people. As the members of the counterculture found themselves ready to settle down and start families, from 1971 to 1980, over 2000 children were born, delivered by the community's midwives.

In 1975, the community published the book Spiritual Midwifery, a collection of birth stories written by the mothers of The Farm, collected and assembled by the midwives.'

Here are some of the birth statistics for The Farm in Tennessee where expectant mums have access to calm, positive birth preparation as standard:

Home births: 94.7%

Caesarean births: 1.7%

Ventouse / forceps extraction: 0.41%

'Hypnobirthing is as much a philosophy of birth as a technique for birthing. It's based on the foundation that all natural, normal functions of the body are achieved without pain.' – Marie Mongan.

What Is The Purpose Of Pain?

When we experience pain, why is that?

What is our body telling us?

When we feel pain in an area of our body, that pain serves as a message telling us to either stop doing something or change the way we are doing it.

Can you think of any times when pain has alerted you of such an issue?

An example that comes up for me when I think about this is when jogging, I have sometimes suddenly been stopped in my tracks by a debilitating pain and seizing up of the calf muscle in my left leg. Whenever that happened, the message was always clear: to continue running would cause further pain and by stopping, the pain would cease. But that pain would also be a reminder to me the next time I went running, after the muscle had healed, to change something about my running technique - maybe the shoes I wore – or to consider running on different terrain.

Our legs contain skeletal muscles which we consciously control and exert effort through to cause them to do what we want them to do. It is also therefore true, that we can remove exertion allowing the muscles to stop working when pain is experienced. You may wonder what this has to do with birth preparation. In the next chapter, I explain about the muscles involved in birthing and the things those muscles have in common with all of the other muscles in the entire human body. I will also explain how those birthing muscles differ.

'Birth is a natural, normal function for women and their babies and therefore women can

safely birth without pain. Just like the bodies of our sister creatures in nature, the bodies of pregnant women instinctively know how to birth.' – Marie Mongan.

If you conjure up an image of other pregnant or birthing mammals, what do you notice is different about them? Do they talk to each other about birthing their young? Do they even think about birth until the time comes? Do they see birth portrayed in the media in a way that might cause them to doubt their ability to birth as nature intended? If a pet dog or cat goes to the vet during pregnancy or birth, this is only ever if a human has intervened.

And yet, just like all other mammals know how to birth their babies, our bodies know exactly how to birth our babies too.

Imagine a female pet cat is pregnant and she notices sensations in her body telling her that her kittens are going to be born soon. Maybe it's a noisy Saturday morning at home – her adult owners are in the lounge watching tv and the three children are playing in different areas of the house being quite boisterous. There doesn't seem to be a quiet, calm place indoors right now for her. She takes herself outside. She knows exactly where she will be comfortable out there. She heads in the direction of the far corner at the bottom of the garden between the fence and the shed. She has made a nest in this spot many times before, unobserved, and out of direct sunlight. It's quiet, warm, comfortably familiar and a safe environment for her. In these conditions her labour continues for some time without interruption.

Imagine that she suddenly senses a smell that alerts her to the fact there's a fox nearby – probably in the garden. Perhaps she can even see the fox. What effects will this have on her labour?

The safety of her kittens is her priority at that time.

Cats usually have an average of four kittens in each litter. However, this can range from one to 12 kittens. If labour continues and her litter is born whilst the fox is in the garden, how will she keep them all safe and away from the fox? Surely the best thing is for them to stay inside of her until it is safe for them in the garden or until she has moved to a safer environment.

In reaction to her alertness and fear, the labouring cat's subconscious mind sends a message of fear to her body – this causes the release of stress hormones which makes her heart beat faster and sends the oxygenated blood from her uterus to her legs, preparing her to 'fight' or 'flee' the danger. Labour will then resume once she feels safe and comfortable again in the knowledge that her litter is no longer at risk.

The above is an example of what happens to all mammals during the fight or flight, survival response.

It makes complete sense to stop labour in that situation. Our own survival and the protection of our unborn babies is paramount and when the body is busy in vital survival mode, everything else has good cause to shut down – including digestion and the birth process. As women, we also have reasons akin to the fox in the cat example. For us, when we are in the car on the way to the birth centre or when we have first arrived at the hospital and have just met the midwife who will be supporting us through our birth experience, our very powerful subconscious mind will be assessing the environment and deciding if this is a place where we are comfortable for our baby to be born and if we are accepting the fact that this midwife (who we may have never met before) is a person we feel relaxed with, and supported by, to allow birth to happen.

Those are very legitimate reasons for our bodies to temporarily slow things down.

Unfortunately, our subconscious minds cannot tell the difference between a real threat and a perceived threat, meaning that other people's stories, the way the media portrays birth, basically everything we have ever heard, seen and learnt about birth, forms our belief system and builds conditioning layers surrounding what birth means for us. We might slow our own labour down in the same way as explained above, but our reasons for doing this could be unwarranted. No one is born with a fear of birth. Why would evolution want us to be scared of something which is necessary in order to continue the human race? Why would we evolve in a way that caused everyone to fear the only way our bodies know of bringing new life?

Our unique, individual experience of life and conditioning – all the information, feelings, thoughts and fears we store - will have an impact on our physiology during labour and birth. The words used by those supporting us throughout our pregnancy, labour and birth and, even more importantly, the words we tell ourselves, will affect our state of mind.

The late Marie Mongan, founder and grandmother of Hypnobirthing, said that birth could be accomplished gently and calmly for the large number of women who are not in a high-risk situation. Marie has left a wonderful legacy of hypnobirthing and because of her work, many thousands of women have experienced calmer, better births and I am sure that she would agree with me now when I say that hypnobirthing can help any woman, and that if a woman is considered high risk during her pregnancy, she will benefit even more from hypnobirthing than a woman who is considered low risk. If a woman has a heart condition, for example, the tools she equips herself with through hypnobirthing will help to keep her heart rate constant – this in turn will also help her to feel calm throughout the birth process.

'Hypnobirthing helps mothers to align with their innate capacity to birth gently, comfortably, powerfully and even joyfully.' – Marie Mongan.

Yes, you can enjoy birth! I don't promise totally pain-free births (though many of my clients have reported not feeling any pain and some have said they didn't feel their surges at all) but I do firmly believe that a comfortable, calm birth is possible for all women who attend a Rose Method Hypnobirthing course and that a woman's experience of birth will be better with hypnobirthing techniques than without them.

I wonder how many low-risk births would have been high-risk without the gift of hypnobirthing and also how many birth experiences would have avoided the high-risk route they took if the mothers had prepared antenatally with hypnobirthing. If birth does become high risk, when a woman brings into her experience the empowered mindset and tools of hypnobirthing, this enables her to feel calm throughout.

I take care of myself and eat healthily during my pregnancy.

Surges.

A hypnobirthing mum learns to embrace her body's innate knowledge of birthing. She knows what to do. That knowledge can be harnessed by peeling away any negative conditioning picked up throughout her life until now. She will learn to relax into her birthing process, working with her body and her baby and relaxing through each of the surges (contractions) as the empowered birthing goddess she is.

In hypnobirthing, the word 'surge' is used to describe a uterine sensation. Why?

The word 'contraction' sounds, to me, very much like something that is being inflicted on a person whereas a 'surge' sounds like something a person does or creates.

To 'contract' means to make smaller and when you are about to birth your baby, I think it's unhelpful to imagine that the parts of the body involved in that process are becoming smaller.

It can be useful to envisage the uterus surging – the word 'surge' has a connotation of power, a force of nature or moving forward.

In fact, here is the Oxford languages definition of the word:

surge:

noun: a sudden powerful forward or upward movement, by a natural force such as the tide. Similar: rush, stream,

flow, swirling.

The similes in that definition make me think of waves. I believe that the sea and a woman's body during labour have so much in common. The sea sometimes appears very calm and still, even though it is often a different story under the surface. The innate knowing body of a calm, labouring woman also appears very still; however, it will be doing just as it needs to during each stage throughout labour. As you will see when we cover Surge Breathing later, the vivid yet simple imagery for one of the Rose Method visualisations is a wave.

A hypnobirthing woman trusts that her body and her baby each knows their job. Trust reduces the amount of tiredness she feels and the length of her labour. When a woman understands the birth process and what her uterus is doing, it is possible for her to believe in her body's power to get her baby out whilst she remains relaxed. When she is relaxed throughout the surges that her uterus creates, she gives her body permission for each surge to happen at its full capacity. She surrenders to her body's power. In doing so, she lets her uterus surge in a way that is just right for her – she allows the sensations to be powerful without resistance. And with no resistance, she enables each surge to occur and complete in less time. Each individual, powerful surge is over more quickly. Fewer surges are required when each surge is more powerful. Therefore, when a woman is relaxed during labour, the duration of labour is likely to be shorter than if she is tense. Fewer, shorter surges will be needed to reach full dilation. A woman will also feel more energy following a relaxed labour and birth than a frantic one.

A natural surge fuelled by oxytocin and the body's innate knowing of what it needs to do, cannot be too strong for you, because it is you.

A woman's body will only give her what she can take. So, when labour begins, just the right amount of oxytocin is released to produce surges that are exactly right for her and her baby. Her body knows how much her body can take and which hormones it needs to release and how much of each of those hormones.

In reaction to the surges and oxytocin release, she'll also release coping hormones – endorphins are the feel-good hormones; relaxin helps the ligaments and muscles of her pelvis loosen and relax; natural tranquilisers assist in calming her mind. As well as all of those, beta-endorphins are also released. Beta endorphins are four times more powerful than morphine! A woman's body releases all of that when she is calm. You see, your body really does have everything you need to get you through labour and birth and it can be a positive, euphoric experience.

A calm response to labour causes those calming birth hormones to be released. Those birth-friendly hormones are antagonistic to catecholamines (stress hormones) meaning that things like adrenaline and cortisol don't stand a chance when the oxytocin and endorphins, etc., are flowing well.

Augmentation (Speeding Up Labour).

Syntocinon (Pitocin in the US) is NOT the same as the naturally produced hormone released during labour, Oxytocin.

Let's break down the word Oxytocin:

Oxy: Oxygenated
Tocin: Birth

Calming. Relaxing. Balancing. Natural. Exactly what the body needs.

Now, look at the word Syntocinon:

Syn: Synthetic Tocin(on): Birth

As women, we release oxytocin when we're making our babies, as we bond with them during pregnancy, when we go through the labour and birth process with our babies and when we feed and cuddle them after they're born.

During the first part of the birth process, the oxytocin causes surges which will open the cervix. This is called the dilation stage. The latent phase of dilation is when a woman's cervix is 0-4cm open. And from 4cm until full dilation (10cm), this is known as the active dilation phase.

As labour progresses, your body will increase the levels of oxytocin being released as long as you are relaxed, and it will continue to release the coping hormones needed in balance with this. The level of coping hormones keeps up with your natural oxytocin levels because your body knows what to do and what you need.

So, what's the difference when a woman consents to having Syntocinon administered to speed up labour?

Augmentation will often cause much stronger surges - that's the intention, right - meet baby sooner? But it can have the opposite effect...

Why?

If a woman agrees to having her labour augmented (sped up with a hormone drip), an artificial, synthetic hormone called Syntocinon (Pitocin in the US) is drip-fed. This will change the physiology of labour.

How do the midwives know how much of the Syntocinon / Pitocin a woman can take when deciding on the levels for the drip. Also, until that point, her body has responded by releasing just the right amount of natural coping hormones required based on the amount of her body's own natural oxytocin being released. However, her body doesn't recognise synthetic hormones in the same way. The intention of augmentation is to cause stronger surges in the uterus than were being experienced immediately before the Syntocinon / Pitocin was administered. However, the coping hormones will likely not match the new levels of surge-producing, artificial hormones. It is therefore common for a woman to request pain relief quite soon after the augmentation process has started. Consider your options and always remember that health care providers require your consent before any intervention or examination is carried out. Remember, you are the expert of yourself and your body. You are also the only person who should decide what, if anything, is done to your body at any time in your life, including during pregnancy, labour and birth.

Your body doesn't recognise Syntocinon in the same way it recognises Oxytocin. The release of coping hormones will slow down in response to the artificial hormone. This can instantly create unmanageable sensations, causing a woman to want something to replace that natural cocktail of support that her amazing body was giving her before. In fact, the sudden artificially-increased intensity will often result in a woman engaging the neo-cortex part of her brain to start thinking. Of course, it is very normal to wonder why things have suddenly become so much more intense. The conscious mind has a natural tendency to question why things have changed so abruptly. It will alert the subconscious part of the mind, which wants to protect us from anything we are frightened of or that causes us pain. This will then cause tension in the uterus muscles. The outermost, longitudinal uterine muscles (running vertically down the uterus) will work less effectively. These muscles need the oxygenated blood to flow well through the uterus's blood vessels, but if a labouring woman begins to panic, then the blood will be directed to her limbs. That's because she is subconsciously sending a message to her body that there is something to fear or a risk to handle, and dangers, fears or risks, whether they are real or perceived, take priority to deal with over birth. So, the body gets ready to run or defend (fight or flight). In fact, if there really was a threat such as suddenly being in a warzone, the womb is likely to be the best place for baby to stay put right now. When the body is getting ready to defend or flee, it will focus on that and only that, therefore releasing hormones to help deal with that immediate need – adrenaline and cortisol. The subconscious mind reacts to how we feel about a situation – the fear response we have in reaction to a stimulus, rather than the actual situation itself. Feeling uncomfortable or anxious when labour starts, will cause the subconscious mind to go into protection mode because it believes it is keeping us safe from danger.

It is at that point when many women request external pain relief options. I'm not against pain relief per se, just when it's a result of being underinformed, in this case, about augmentation.

Your body knows what to do during labour

to bring your baby to you...

just like the sea knows exactly what to do to bring the waves to the shore.

Trust your body...

Trust birth...

You've got this!

My cervix dilates gradually just as nature intended, and my birth path opens in its own perfect time.

In Tune With Your Body And Your Baby.

Another advantage of being calm during labour and birth is that you will be in tune with what your body is feeling. You will get used to how the sensations of labour feel in the body and those sensations will be unhindered because of your relaxed state. If something suddenly feels different or not quite right, you will be aware of those changes and notice anything unusual. Remember, like I said before, you know your own body better than anyone else and you are the expert of yourself and your body so, in fact, you are likely going to be able to highlight any concerns you might have, often before the midwife, doctor or anyone else who is observing your labour notices. However, when a woman is in a nervous or panicked state of mind during labour, because of the affect that has on her body, especially the uterus, she is unlikely to detect any slight changes in the sensations because they feel like part and parcel of the feelings she was already experiencing which were brought about by her fight or flight response to the labour.

The late Marie Mongan's own birth experiences led her to develop the first ever hypnobirthing program. Marie was the original founder of hypnobirthing and also a hypnobirthing grandmother.

Marie gave birth to her first child in 1955. She discarded all negative literature about childbirth and focussed on Grantly Dick-Read's theory of eliminating the 'Fear-Tension-Pain' syndrome.

All of Marie's labours were calm and relaxed.

During her first birth experience, hospital staff didn't believe she could have been in advanced labour and so left her unattended. She called the nurses when the baby was crowning and even though she was ready to give birth precisely there and then and she and her baby were safe and in no danger, the nurses pushed her legs together and told her she must wait because she wasn't in the delivery room yet.

Once in the room deemed appropriate, they forced an ether cone onto Marie's face and her baby was hurried out by forceps.

This type of birth was common-place and normality in that era and the birth of Marie's second child was very similar to the first.

We are very lucky though that Marie fought hard for what she believed in, and that she went on to have two more children. For her younger two children's births went just as she had wished (after much confrontation with her doctor) and she was the talk of the hospital following both. There was no unnecessary intervention as there was with the first two. Unfortunately, people were sceptical after the initial novelty and excitement wore off and they began to say that she merely had a very high pain threshold and her births were quickly dismissed as a fluke.

Marie didn't give up though! She went on to train as a hypnotherapist and developed the HypnoBirthing programme when her daughter was pregnant. The very first Hypnobirthing baby was therefore Marie's first grandchild.

I must reiterate that Marie achieved this against all odds at a time when there was no internet. She did it on her own without a practitioner, just by believing in herself and in the miracle of Mother Nature. And if she could do that then at a time when very few women were having births like that in developed countries, you can do it now!

My birth experience is not the sum of other people's birth stories. My birth experience is created by me – by my body – by my mind – by my baby

HOUR TWO

The Uterus

I have mentioned the uterine muscles a few times already. It's time to explain a lot more about the amazing organ that is the uterus.

The uterus is a smooth muscle. It is an involuntary muscle. Smooth, involuntary muscles are found within the walls of organs and structures such as the oesophagus, stomach, intestines, bronchi, bladder, blood vessels which pump oxygenated blood all over the body for us, the arrector pili in the skin (this controls when your hair stands on end and causes the goosebump response – on your forearm for example).

Unlike skeletal muscle, which is under conscious control, we cannot consciously control smooth muscle. To explain this, imagine if you wanted to lift a heavy object, you would engage your biceps and exert effort to pick the object up. When your biceps are working to give you the strength needed to do that, your triceps relax. For every action on one side of a muscle group, if the muscle group is going to work as was intended, there needs to be an opposing reaction on the other side of that muscle group. So, one side of the muscle is active whilst the other side is passive. That will be useful to bear in mind shortly as you read on.

But, before I move on, did you know that, as well as being a growing organ where your baby is developing, the uterus is also the strongest muscle group in the entire human body.

Your uterus is so strong that women in comas have given birth vaginally without any assistance.

Being in a coma means that a person's mind is sleeping. Their body continues to function as do their reproductive organs. The baby would also continue to develop and when the right time came, the body would prepare itself for birthing.

That's exactly what happened in 2001, when doctors in Cincinnati learned a patient named Chastity Cooper was two weeks pregnant when she suffered serious head injuries in a car accident and lapsed into a coma. The pregnancy was carried to term and delivered vaginally, as doctors ruled out a C-section because of the risks of giving anaesthesia to comatose patients. (source: rollingstone.com website).

How can it possibly be that this set of muscles is the strongest in the entire human body, is carrying out one of the most vital of actions – bringing new life into the world, and yet it seems to be the one that does not function correctly and which we hear so many negative, traumatic stories about?

Shouldn't the birthing muscles perform naturally and just as efficiently as all of the other muscles in the body do?

When we use our other muscles, do they hurt at the time of exertion? Aren't they more likely to experience discomfort the next day or even a couple of days later?

In fact, DOMS (delayed onset of muscle soreness) is common when we use any muscles a bit more than usual. The morning after giving birth to my daughter, I woke to the slight, quiet sound of her communicating to me that she was hungry. We were in the postnatal ward and throughout the night, three other mums and newborns had joined us in the room so I wanted to be quick in reaching for Orla to prevent her from resorting to crying louder as that would likely have woken everyone else in the room. So, I sat up and leant forward and as I did, it felt like I had done about 150 sit-ups the day before and that I hadn't done any for about a year. DOMS after labour - of course, it makes complete sense because the uterus is like all other muscles, in that it's performing a natural, normal, expected, automatic function which it is designed specifically to do. But I didn't know until it happened to me.

During your first hypnobirthing class, it will be explained to you how the uterus is made up and you will be shown the window to the womb drawings on the next few pages.

When your practitioner asked you what the job of your longitudinal uterus muscles are during pregnancy, did you guess or did you know? And did you know what the other 2 muscle layers are responsible for as well or was that easier to answer once the outer layer was explained to you? Most people will go through pregnancy, labour and birth without knowing very much about the uterus muscles at all. But I think it can make a huge difference to the way we feel about undergoing a process if we know what is going to happen during that process. And this is why everyone who comes to me for a hypnobirthing course, practitioner training or even a taster session will learn what the muscles of the uterus do during pregnancy, what they do during labour and what they do during birth and how the mind and our thoughts and beliefs can and will profoundly affect the process.

The longitudinal muscle fibres are the muscles closest to the surface of the uterine walls and they run up and down the uterus. During pregnancy they are passive.

The middle muscle layer contains muscle fibres, and their job is to pump the optimum amount of oxygenated blood around the uterus for you and your baby at all times during pregnancy, labour and birth. This encourages the release of oxytocin – your fuel for a calm birth. Oxytocin literally means 'oxygen birth'.

The innermost, circular muscle layer contains muscle fibres that run across the uterus horizontally and which are more concentrated towards the lowest part of the uterus near the cervix. During pregnancy they are active when their job is to keep everything as it is. I often say that these particular muscles are shaped like a cradle, holding everything in and supporting the baby.

The above happens all by itself because a woman's body knows exactly what it needs to do at each stage of growing her baby and your body also knows exactly what to do to bring him or her into the world. At the start of your Hypnobirthing course, your practitioner might have asked you if you ever need to exert any effort to make the above happen. Of course, you don't have to. And the reason you don't have to is because the uterus contains smooth, involuntary muscles. Women don't really think about this part of the process – we take for granted how it just happens. However, many women do worry about what will happen once labour starts.

By the way, if you do sometimes feel a sensation in the lower abdominal area during pregnancy, for example, when stepping out of the car after a long journey, getting up from a low sofa or even turning over in your sleep at night, this is likely your circular uterine muscles re-adjusting as you change position.

Then, when a woman goes into labour, what happens to the different uterine muscle layers?

A lot of you will have said at this point during your hypnobirthing class, 'They switch / swap / do the opposite,' and that is correct.

The outer, longitudinal muscles become active and the oxygenated blood continues to flow well around the uterus's blood vessels even more now that the body's resources can focus away from other functions and focus on the birth process and bringing your baby to you.

And the circular muscles need to relax for labour to feel comfortable and for the muscles to work efficiently together. They need to be passive whenever the longitudinal layer is active.

The surge of the longitudinal muscles draws up, flexes, and expels; the lower horizontal muscles relax to allow birth to happen. This is the set of muscles working in harmony just as nature intended. It is also important to remember that both parts of the uterine muscles also need the middle muscle layer to pump just the right amount of oxygenated blood around the uterus as this makes all the difference and facilitates the working of the other parts of the uterus muscle. The cervix thins and opens, and birthing occurs smoothly and easily.

A Window To The Womb.

Longitudinal Muscles

The longitudinal muscle fibres are the muscles closest to the surface of the uterine walls and they run up and down the uterus. During pregnancy they are passive. When labour begins, they become active by drawing up, flexing, and expelling. Drawing on the opposite page.

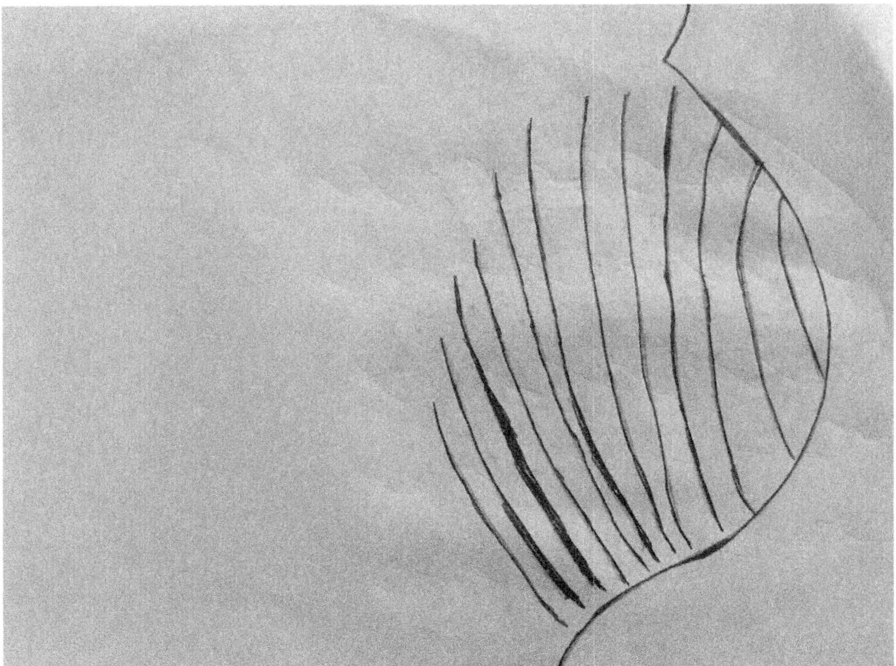

Middle Muscle Layer

The middle muscle layer consists of muscle fibres whose job it is to pump the optimum amount of oxygenated blood around the uterus for you and your baby at all times during pregnancy, labour and birth. This further encourages the release of oxytocin – your fuel for a calm birth. Oxytocin literally means oxygen birth. Drawing on the opposite page.

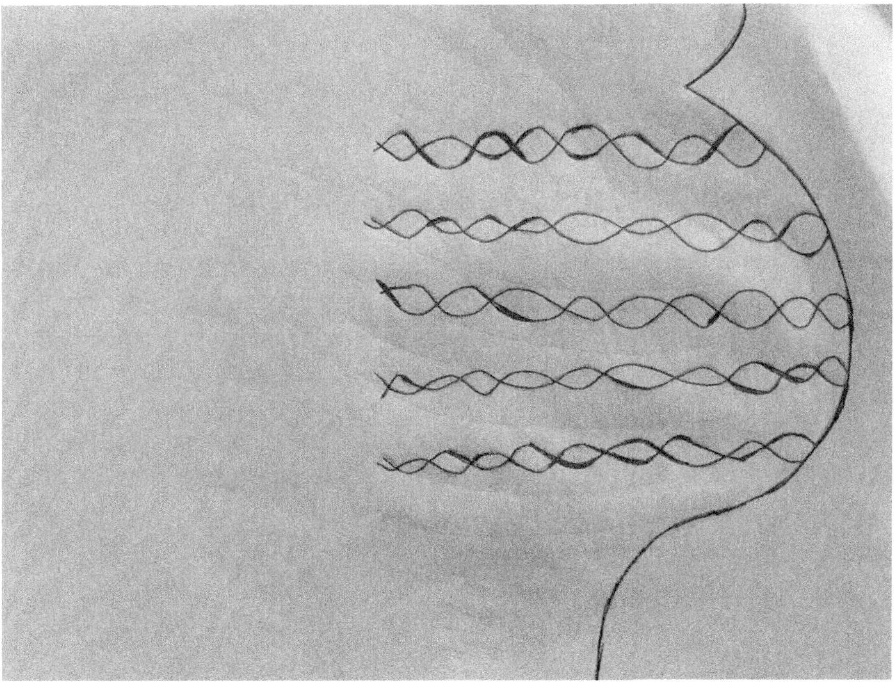

Horizontal Muscles

The innermost, circular, cradle-shaped muscle fibres run across the uterus horizontally. They are more concentrated towards the lowest part of the uterus near the cervix. During pregnancy, they are active when their job is to keep everything as it is. During labour and birth, in order for labour to feel comfortable and for the uterine muscles as a whole to be efficient, these circular muscles need to be passive and relaxed to allow birth to happen. Drawing on the opposite page.

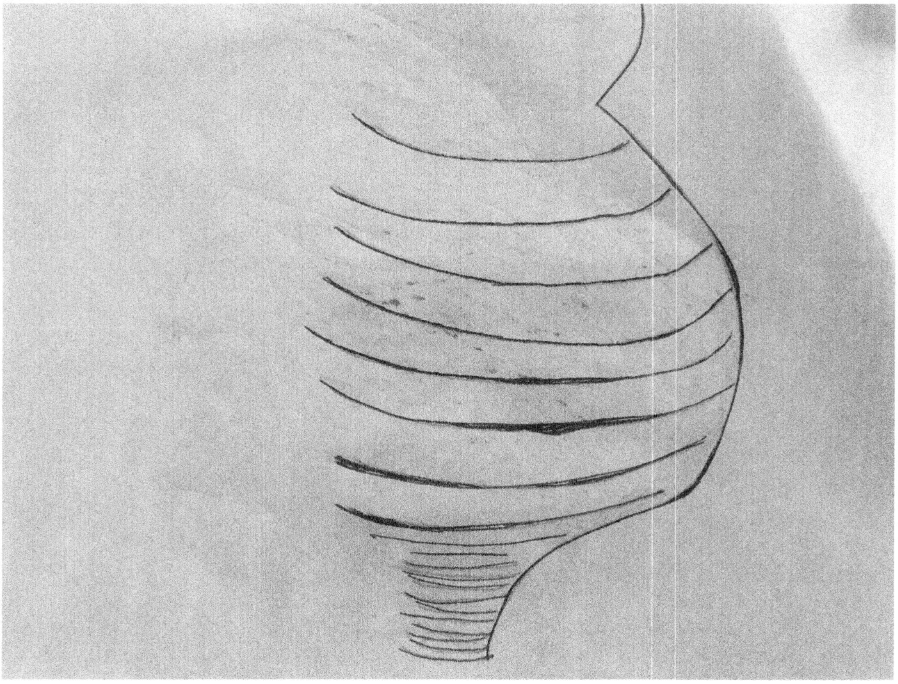

Baby In Utero

Your baby is in the amniotic fluid of the uterus and the umbilical cord connects the baby to the placenta. Drawing on opposite page.

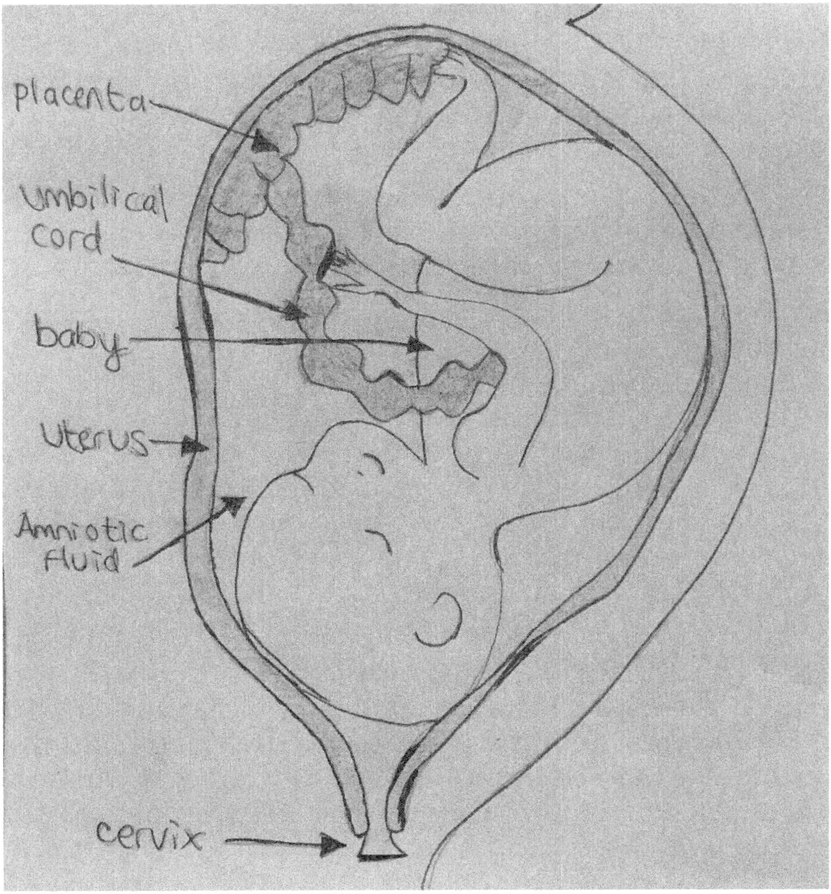
placenta
umbilical cord
baby
Uterus
Amniotic fluid
cervix

Why does labour hurt so much for so many women?

Did you already know about the 'fight or flight' response before you started to learn about birth and did you think that it was a factor that caused pain during labour; pain which for a lot of women could have been minimised or even eliminated had labour been preceded by good antenatal preparation. Most of the women who attend my classes have never been told how their uterus muscles are made up until they come to my first session or until they read this book. They have never been told that their expectations and beliefs about labour and birth will impact how those muscles work when their surges start.

If tension exists during labour, the longitudinal outer muscles will do their job less effectively. These muscles need the oxygenated blood to flow well through the uterus's blood vessels (middle layer) but if a woman is fearful during labour, then the blood will be directed where?

When a woman panics during labour, the oxygenated blood is directed to her arms and legs as they are part of her defence mechanism and of course the muscles of the uterus are not.

With the oxygenated blood being pumped to other parts of the body during labour, the circular muscles running across the uterus tense up again instead of relaxing as they need to at that time, and the longitudinal muscles are still working but less effectively. Both sides of the uterus muscle working at the same time is akin to engaging our biceps and triceps simultaneously which would cause the upper arm to go into spasm. Remember, for every action on one side of a muscle group, there needs to be an opposing reaction on the other side of that muscle group for the body to work as nature intends it to. Otherwise, the muscle group will experience spasm, cramp, and pain.

The very powerful subconscious part of our minds is always looking to protect us and it reacts to how something makes us feel rather than being able to look objectively at whether or not we need protection. This is because the subconscious mind is unable to differentiate between a real threat and a perceived threat.

Stress causes and contributes to 90% of all disease (unease / dis-ease manifests as disease and physical pain) so why wouldn't that also be the case during pregnancy and labour? Our stresses, our fears, our karma or conditioning, whatever term you want to use for it, causes us to experience a different physiology in the body, the fight or flight response, releasing catecholamines or stress hormones like cortisol, adrenaline, etc… Those hormones are antagonistic to the birth hormones.

'Unfamiliar people in birthing rooms, bright lights and certain words or phrases will alter the chemistry of any woman's body during labour. Stress can sneak in and disrupt mum and baby's physiology and well-being during labour, often leading to complications.' – Marie Mongan.

I'll say it again because it is important: catecholamines and oxytocin are antagonistic – they cannot co-exist. Stress creates a constriction of blood vessels, thus reducing the amount of oxygen for the labouring mum and her baby. It creates irregular surges, prevents labour from progressing or even from starting in the first place and can stop the cervix from opening.

But why are many women in our society so frightened of birth? I know I was, and I know a lot of the ladies I have taught hypnobirthing to came to me because they were. But why?

Like I have said before, no one is born into this world with a fear of birth programmed into them. People will form their opinion of how they think labour and birth is or how it will feel for them. They build what is often an exaggerated picture of birth from tv programmes, news articles, stories they've heard from well-intentioned friends, stories they've overheard on the bus to work, the views of those in an assumed position of expertise and / or authority, what we are taught in school about birth, etc. We are not born with a fear of birth, and we can peel away the unhelpful layering and conditioning.

'The autonomic nervous system is the communication network within our bodies. It interprets messages and determines which action should be taken as a result of each message. Our nervous system takes us to the sympathetic part of the autonomic nervous system when we feel threatened by something or someone.' – Marie Mongan.

And remember, the subconscious responds in exactly the same way to perceived threats as it does to real threats. We know if we're crossing the road and, suddenly realise that a vehicle is moving towards us a lot faster than we had thought it was, that we need to get across the road fast! Catecholamines (stress hormones) are released to make our hearts race faster to enable the oxygen to be directed quickly where we need it to be if we are going to run or defend ourselves. The subconscious doesn't know the reason for the fear – it responds to whatever we are feeling at that given time.

These moments of fight or flight put us into survival mode

briefly. But when there is a real emergency, that is the exact response we need. As soon as the immediate risk has been averted, the blood in our bodies starts to flow all around again, our heart returns to its resting rate. We are no longer panicking. We are feeling calm once more.

Now, if a woman has heard lots of negative messages about birth throughout her life, those negative messages are likely to have been accepted as true by her subconscious mind and they become part of her belief system. So, when that same woman goes into labour, her very powerful subconscious mind believes that it needs to provide a protective role. It sends messages of fear via the autonomic nervous system and the same thing happens as if there is a real threat.

The situation the woman is in is seen, by her mind, as a dangerous one requiring defence mechanisms and of course the uterus is not part of the defence mechanism. Therefore, oxygenated blood is directed away from it to the arms and legs.

'This limits the amount of oxygen getting to the baby. With limited oxygen and blood, the lower circular muscles in the uterus constrict and tighten. That is, of course, the complete opposite of what they are made to do. Instead of relaxing as it needs to, the cervix remains taut and closed. The baby's head then pushes against circular uterus

muscles which are not yet relaxed and open enough to accommodate it. This is then often described by the medical profession as 'Failure to Progress' which has coincidentally got the same three initials as Fer-Tension-Pain which Grantly Dick-Read described in his book 'Childbirth without Fear', as the reason for pain in childbirth for otherwise healthy women. Pain is then created, and labour is prolonged. The opening of the cervix is impeded. Then intervention is often introduced to 'rescue' mum and baby but of course the fear that caused the pain and slow progress was unwarranted anyway.' – Marie Mongan.

I trust myself and my own pregnancy, labour, birth, and parenting choices.

HOUR THREE

It doesn't have to be like that - how to have a calm birth.

On the other hand, is the parasympathetic part of the autonomic nervous system (the ANS). This is what keeps the body and mind in a state of harmony and balance. When we are totally calm, relaxed and at ease, this is where we go. Endorphins exist here and shut out the enemy hormone of the birth room – catecholamine.

Learning how to get yourself into a calm state of mind and to feel comfortable and relaxed in your body and then to maintain those feelings (and bring yourself back to those feelings if there are any distractions such as thoughts, people, change to the environment) is a big part of what Hypnobirthing is. Learning about what your body will do during labour is the first part of this because, when we are aware of what our body is going to do, we are better able to trust the process, trust our bodies and trust our babies to do what they need to do.

Now that you know how the muscles of the uterus work during pregnancy and labour, let's talk about how to get and keep women in this 'healing room' - the parasympathetic part of the ANS during labour and birth.

'What labour needs is more awareness of the importance of calm, the importance of relaxation and some gentle encouragement and assurance

should be given to a labouring woman to enable labour to move along at her pace.

Rather than cure with pain relief, the aim should be to prevent pain.' –Hypnobirthing - The Mongan Method.

Birth partners, midwives, doctors and anyone else present, would do well to speak encouragingly and kindly to a labouring woman during labour. If she chooses to be examined the first time she sees a midwife during her labour, whether she is told that her cervix is 3cm, 5cm or 8cm dilated, be mindful of the words used. Words like 'only', 'just', 'not much' have no place here. More helpful things to say are, 'already', 'halfway', 'doing so well', 'almost'.

I agreed to a vaginal examination when I first arrived at the birth centre mainly because hypnobirthing was not a concept the midwives who had been assigned to me were familiar with and after my surges had reduced from being three minutes apart when we left home to seven minutes apart en route, and I may have appeared less advanced into my labour than I actually was. I heard whispers like, 'I think we're going to have to send this one home'. And then one of the midwives asked me if that was me having a contraction as I stood still and leant against the corridor wall for some support when we were walking from the entrance of the maternity unit to the midwife led area (The Haven Birthing Suite at Poole).

The idea of having an examination to see how labour is progressing, appeals to some women and you deserve to be respected whether you want to be examined or not. That is your choice because it's your body and your birth experience. However, knowing how far your cervix has opened at any given time is no indication of when your baby will be born. In my case, I was concerned about being sent home if they had no measurable way to ascertain that I was in established labour already. Yes, it would have been great if they trusted me to know my own body and I will say that this was 2007 and that since then, midwives are a lot more familiar with hypnobirthing.

I will always remember the look of shock on the midwife's face as she examined me. She was down the business end and then suddenly looked up at my face and said, 'Bloody hell, you're 8cm dilated – you'll have a baby by lunchtime!' She then held my hand and said how sorry she was for not believing that I was ready to be there and explained that it was because they were not used to seeing women as calm as I was in established labour – let alone at 8 cm dilated.

'Keep doing whatever it is you have been doing,' she said.

To be honest, the encouragement and assurance was just what I needed but I look back now and think it was a shame it took the shock of seeing a woman calmly labouring when 8cm dilated to receive such supportive comments. What does that tell us about the way a woman is expected to look when she is in established labour? Isn't that sad?

Always remember too, that your consent is necessary before a midwife or doctor examines you or intervenes in any way during your labour, for it is your body they would be examining.

During the first session of your course, I expect you will have seen a hypnobirth film or maybe your practitioner has shared a YouTube link of one for you to watch in your own time. Hopefully you will have the chance to see one birth at each of your sessions – these are births that are not available to watch on the internet. If you are given suggestions of births to watch at home, I would recommend you watch those too – ideally after playing a relaxation MP3. You'll notice that your practitioner will wait until immediately after a relaxation exercise you do in class before showing a birth film. This is because, after having experienced a deep state of relaxation, your mind will absorb and retain the positive images you see on the inspiring birth film better than if you watch it when your mind is very busy. I hope you enjoyed a relaxation exercise during which you also learnt one of the Rose Method hypnobirthing breathing techniques – I call this first breathing technique Esdaille Resting Breaths – the breathing technique you might like to use during the rest times between your surges. It's great to have a breathing technique to focus on during those times to prevent the mind from thinking about the previous surge and worrying about the next one. The breathing technique works together with an anchoring word – usually 'Lavender', but you can change this to something else if you like. The script is my own version of an adaptation Marie Mongan wrote of James Esdaille's script which, because of its pacing, use of words and technique is thought to help those hearing it to reach a trance like state that some have described as a hypnotic coma. It enables the listener to experience a feeling close to delta (sleep).

How wonderful would it be to feel that way between the surges, thereby conserving your energy?

HOMEWORK

- Between now and the next time you meet with your practitioner, I would recommend taking some time to practise your Esdaille Resting Breaths.
- Another good idea is to read until the end of this page after your first session. Stop here and enjoy the next part of the book after your next session.
- Now is also a great time to download your MP3s if you haven't already:
    - Aurora Relaxation for Birth – great to play as you are ready to drift off to sleep each night. Ideally you will fall asleep as it is playing, as this will open the gateway from the conscious to the subconscious part of your mind and enable all of the positivity to be absorbed and to help you feel calm and confident about your upcoming birth.
    - Words of Conscious Re-Affirmation – the best time to play this is when you are getting ready for the day ahead (for example, when you're having your breakfast). I refer to these statements as reaffirming because you were born with the innate wisdom they hold – you just need reminding of them. After

hearing the Conscious Reaffirming MP3 a few times, you might have several favourite affirmations. It's a good idea to write those down on some coloured post-its and to pop those in prominent places around the home where you will regularly see them (next to the bed, on the kettle, on the fridge, around your pc or laptop screen etc). It's a good idea to rotate the post-its occasionally too. On the next page follows the full Re-Affirmations in case if you would like to read them to yourself too.

Words Of Conscious Re-Affirmation

My birth experience is not the sum of other people's birth stories. My birth experience is created by me – by my body – by my mind – by my baby.

I trust myself and my own pregnancy, labour, birth and parenting choices.

I trust each stage of the birth process.

My surroundings and the people supporting me keep me calm and really relaxed throughout my labour and birth.

I choose to enjoy birth.

By learning about birth and practising my relaxation techniques, I get to create a calm, empowered internal environment and inner voice on the lead up to and during the time my baby is born.

When I am calm and comfortable during pregnancy and birth, my baby is calm and comfortable too.

I trust that my body knows exactly what to do to make, grow and bring my baby to me.

I stop unnecessary interference by relaxing my conscious mind.

I trust my body and the process of giving birth.

My uterus is the strongest part of me; it knows what to do and it works in harmony with nature.

My birthing body does everything at exactly the right pace for me and for my baby.

I am the expert of my body.

My cervix dilates gradually just as nature intended and my birth path opens in its own perfect time.

I give myself permission to surrender to the power of my birthing body.

My body is making way, perfectly, for my baby's journey.

I take care of myself and eat healthily during my pregnancy.

My body is healthy and grows my baby to a healthy size that I can give birth to.

I breathe slowly and visualise throughout my powerful surges.

I am everything that I need to be and more, to make, grow, welcome and parent my baby.

I breathe as my uterus rises and nudges my baby down to meet me.

My uterus relaxes between surges to give my baby the time and space needed to move down.

I imagine that my placenta detaches and emerges easily.

I look forward to meeting and holding my baby, their skin to my skin.

I trust each stage of the birth process.

HOUR FOUR

When you start reading this chapter, you have likely completed six hours of classes with your practitioner. Your recap reading will be from here until the end of Hour Six. I hope you are thoroughly enjoying your classes so far, feel supported by your practitioner and confident about your pregnancy, labour and birth journey. I love hearing from anyone learning The Rose Method so do drop me a line if you'd like to.

At the beginning of this session, I expect you enjoyed a relaxation exercise before watching a non-waterbirth. A lot of the hypnobirths that are available to watch online or that Hypnobirthing mums have said they are happy for practitioners to show during classes, are waterbirths and I think there are two reasons for this. Women mainly see waterbirths in their hypnobirthing classes and then opt for a waterbirth themselves because of how calm the women look in the videos. I also think there are less non-water hypnobirth films available to see as women feel more comfortable sharing their birth for others to be inspired by, when they are modestly covered by the water. I remain so very grateful to all of the ladies who have shared their birth videos, so that we can continue to inspire others with real examples of how hypnobirthing makes for a calm birth. I wonder, will you be filming your birth – to keep for yourself and your baby or to share and inspire others? Your baby's birth is such an intimate, private event in your life and so it is completely your choice, but I would be delighted to hear from you if you do decide to film it and would be ok with future Rose Method clients seeing it during classes.

Watching calm birth films during your hypnobirthing course will help you to replace any images which might cause you to feel some fear around going into labour.

Anchors

Have you given any thought to what you might use to set up an environment conducive to relaxation during labour and birth? What would serve as tangible anchors to bring you back to a feeling of comfort in case anything distracts you or decreases your level of relaxation at any time during your labour?

We naturally anchor our emotions through our senses, and we use different senses for each type of anchor. Some people are more visual whilst others are more auditory - affected more by sounds and music. Do you know which modality you are?

Olfactory

The feelings that a certain smell evokes can transfer a person to a place or time that the smell reminds them of. For example, whenever I smell the subtle scent of vanilla, I am often transported in my mind to the kitchen of my late grandparents. Whenever I visited them as a young girl, there was always a distinct smell and I probably wasn't really aware of what it was at the time, but Nana was often baking and I am reminded of her handing me the mixing bowl and wooden spoon to give her Victoria sandwich ingredients a stir, the yellow and brown kitchen tiles and the larder. Whenever I smell vanilla nowadays, it's so very reminiscent of my nana in her kitchen.

If you have a favourite smell that you like and that relaxes and comforts you during your practice, you will be able to start building an associated link between that smell and your relaxation. If you have a scented candle that you really like and that helps you to feel calm at home, it's a good idea to find a room spray with that same aroma. Unfortunately, naked flames are not allowed in birth centres and hospitals, but the room spray combined with battery-operated tealights dotted around the room is a good alternative. Plug-in and reed-diffusers work well too. The important thing, if you plan to spend some of your labour or birth in hospital, is to mask any typical hospital smells – often the smell of a hospital evokes feelings of being in a place where people go when they are unwell. You have the opportunity to prevent or reduce those feelings.

An anchor can be learnt by practising and building an associated link to how relaxing something is. During a hypnobirth, it's a great idea to appeal to all of the senses so that if one of the senses is disturbed (for example if the music suddenly stops in the birthing environment because your device needs charging) then you still have other anchors to keep you calm and really relaxed. If you were just depending on the music playing on that particular device for your serene state of mind, then what would happen if that suddenly stopped?

As a side note, it's worth considering playing your music through headphones but then to also play the same or similar music in the room so that everyone else is on the same page as you. This is good as your partner and the health professionals will be better able to calmly support you if they are experiencing the same, calm environment as you are.

The door sign

The Hypnobirthing door sign, which your practitioner has hopefully already given you to put up outside your room if you are planning to give birth in a birth centre or a hospital, is a useful reminder to midwives, when they enter your room, that it is a calm space and that they are mindful of the type of experience you want to have and their natural response is to speak calmly and gently to you so they are contributing positively towards this desired environment. They will love coming into your birthing environment. It's possible that no one else they've supported, in recent days, will have set up their birthing space in a way that's conducive to having a relaxed birth experience. I think that a midwife's job must be really rewarding anyway but that when the woman she is supporting is calm and relaxed, it must feel like a joy to be there compared with if the labouring mum is panicking, fearful and out of control. Hypnobirths are amazing to witness and support.

Relaxed hands

Some of our relaxation techniques are delivered through touch and a very simple technique is 'Relaxed Hands' which I am sure you have already experienced or seen being demonstrated during your recent hypnobirthing class. Women can practise and use this by themselves. It is only possible to do the Relaxed Hands technique when your hands are loosely interlinked, meaning that it is a great, dual-purpose relaxation technique. It has the effect of being calming and also prevents us from tightening up or tensing the muscles in our hands. It can feel tempting to hold onto handles (for example in a birth pool) just to have something to do with our hands and when we do this, we are activating those muscles which sends a message to the blood vessels in our body to pump oxygenated blood from wherever it is in abundance at that time (hopefully the uterus) all the way up through our torso and along our arms, into our hands to our fingertips – it's about the furthest distance it ever needs to travel. Does a woman's oxygenated blood ever need to be there during labour? Under what circumstances when your body is bringing your baby to you, would it be beneficial to send the oxygenated blood from the part of the body that works the hardest during labour and birth to the part that helps us to run away or defend ourselves? Surely, the only time that would be beneficial is if a situation occurred which meant that the baby was safer inside the uterus. Having relaxed hands is a good thing during labour.

Technique: With loosely interlinked fingers, begin to stroke one thumb with the other, up from the base of the thumb very slowly towards the nail. After several strokes, whilst keeping the hands as they are, stop and slowly switch so that the thumb that was being stroked is now stroking the other thumb. It may feel more sensitive when you switch. A slight modification to this technique is to roll the thumbs around each other in circles very slowly in a way that they are barely touching (a gentle, slow version of twiddling your thumbs). Being aware of this simple but effective way to keep your hands calm and relaxed, can act as a great reminder to think before tensing, grabbing, or gripping during labour and birth.

Lighting

Practising your relaxation in a dark or dimly lit room is a good idea as most people relax better in dim lighting as we are used to sleeping with little or no light. You can then make the space in which you labour and birth in a similar amount of light as you're used to practising in. Dimming the lights at home and / or in the birth centre is a great idea, as is a string of battery-operated fairy lights in jars or vases or draped across the room. Battery-operated tealights and candles are wonderful for creating an environment that encourages oxytocin release.

My favourite device for creating a gorgeous choice of colour & lighting together with the emission of whatever smell you choose is an Innogear electric diffuser. Just fill with water and a few drops of your chosen oil & set to whichever colour you like or leave it to work through all the colours – it's beautiful and calming. www.innogear.com

My surroundings and the people supporting me keep me calm and really relaxed throughout my labour and birth.

HOUR FIVE

Soothing strokes

Soft, soothing strokes cleverly overwhelm the sensory system, safely and comfortably making changes to the electrical activity in our brains.

The central nervous system consists of the brain and the spinal cord which means that the nerves in our backs are particularly sensitive. Therefore, when a repetitive, soft soothing stroke is applied simultaneously on both sides of the spine, a message of pleasurable feelings is sent from the brain to the skin and to other places in our bodies that are regulated by our central nervous system. This is an excellent example of how every action is triggered by a message sent from the mind to the body – otherwise known as the psycho-physical.

It is not the artificial suppression of symptoms which is experienced when soft soothing strokes are applied. This is a real physical response experienced in the body.

It has been compared with a TENS machine, but the approaches are very different.

A soft, soothing stroke is physical touch from another person – usually your birth partner – that enhances the sensations and experience of labour by naturally stimulating and causing the release of hormones that make us feel good. Whereas the intention of a TENS is to partially block the sensations.

A TENS (transcutaneous electrical nerve stimulation) machine is a small, battery-operated device that connects adhesive electrodes to a device via individual wires. When switched on, tingling sensations will be felt as small electrical impulses are delivered to the area of the body where the electrodes are attached. The impulses can relieve pain by blocking some of the messages sent from the brain to the body.

You can use a TENS machine if you'd like to and it does help a lot of women in labour. If you do use one, then you can still benefit from some soft, soothing strokes on the upper part of your back and shoulders whilst the TENS pads are on your lower back.

Is a TENS machine an anchor?

Would you practise using a TENS machine during pregnancy, thereby building an associated link between that and your relaxation? No. When a woman benefits from a TENS machine, the first time it's used is during labour.

Do soft, soothing strokes act as an anchor?

Hell, yes! Many of my hypnobirthing clients have practised soft, soothing strokes weekly or even daily together with their birth partner to build an associated link between the soothing strokes and their relaxation so that by the time they receive these feather touches during labour, the strokes act as an anchor, their partner's touch is also an anchor and partners can add the use of prompt words together with the soft, soothing strokes to combine the feeling of touch with the sound of their voice.

During practice, until 37 weeks, the soft, soothing strokes should only be enjoyed on the back area as demonstrated by your practitioner during class. However, from 37 weeks and / or during labour, if your partner also strokes your hair, extend their hands out to your ears, face, the front of your neck and décolletage, the sides of your breasts, then as well as the endorphins being produced by touching the back area in such a specific way, a natural oxytocin is created and that powerful cocktail of hormones can encourage strong, effective surges when the touch is enjoyable for you. There will be some anchors and techniques that you like and other that you find less enjoyable which is another reason for practising during pregnancy rather than waiting to see what works once you're already in labour.

Soft, soothing strokes are just one of the many ways birth partners can help during labour.

Certain words can also act as an anchor during labour and birth. Other words can be triggering. This is why the word 'sensation' might sound more positive than the word 'pain' and the word 'surge' more empowering to a woman than the word 'contraction'. The definition of the word 'contraction' is to become smaller. A surge sounds so much more powerful - something amazing that you are doing rather than something that is being inflicted on you.

I hope you also enjoyed the Mongan Method Birth Companion's Exercise during your class. You'll notice that at the end of this chapter, I've strongly recommended practising this together as part of your homework before your next session.

Orla's anchor

About halfway through my pregnancy, my parents found, in their loft, the lovely old crib that I had slept in when I was a baby and that my brother had also slept in when he was a baby. The crib was 35 years old. We ordered a new made-to-measure mattress for it and attached a mobile of soft animal figures friends had gifted us and which we hung over the top. It played lullaby music when we wound it up.

The crib was on my side of the bed and each night, when I was ready to go to sleep, I would stand next to the crib with my bump protruding somewhere between the mobile figurines as they danced around and the mattress of the crib. Then I would wind up the mobile and the lullaby would play for a few minutes. When I think of that time now, I realise that I was playing my baby her relaxation music before playing my own Mongan Method Relaxation each night. This became part of my maternal bedtime routine and after she was born, Orla always seemed soothed by that lullaby as though she recognised it from her time in the womb. This is another example of an anchor!

I choose to enjoy birth

HOUR SIX

Surge breathing

When the uterus is in surge, it rises which re-affirms how very strong the uterus muscles are.

This natural rising of the uterus does not come about through any special breathing technique – a labouring woman's body does this instinctively and very powerfully because it knows it to be the right thing to do.

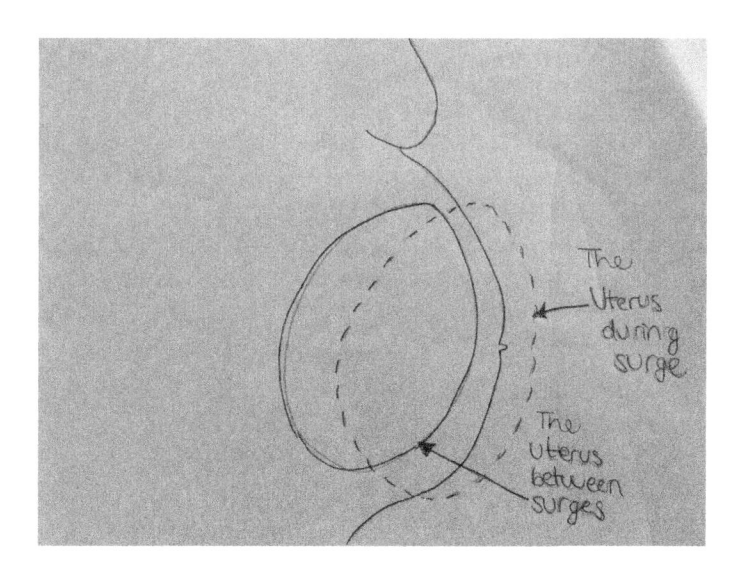

The uterus during surge

The uterus between surges

Essential birth partner reading >>>

Why is it good that this rising of the uterus during each surge is visible to others around the labouring woman at the time?

At home, before leaving for the birth centre or until the home birth midwife arrives, it shows the birth partner when she is having a surge and when she is not. There will be certain things a woman will find comforting and helpful during the rest times, and she may not appreciate those things during a surge. There may also be things that feel very supportive during a surge – for example something a partner might say or do to remind her what to focus on during the surges in order to remain calm.

As a birth partner, you will time the gaps between the surges. Seeing the uterus rise can help with this. The time to measure is from the end of one surge until the beginning of the next. If you are a birth partner, there will be other signals you will start to notice that will help you to differentiate between how your partner appears when she is having a surge and when she is between surges.

- The uterus rises during a surge.
- Your partner's eyes will probably be closed during a surge, or she may appear to be in a more dreamlike state than at other times.
- Another indication is that the rise and fall of the chest will be different during surge breathing than at other times.

It's good to start timing the gaps in between from the beginning of labour so that if your partner needs your support in other ways as labour progresses and the surges may become more intense, you're able to introduce that support when already being used to timing the surges – this is really helpful, supportive multi-tasking. <<< **Essential birth partner reading**

To relax, it is helpful to divert the conscious mind away from thoughts of what is actually happening – not because what is happening is bad – what the body is doing is exactly what it needs to – but when you relax, you connect with the subconscious part of your mind and this allows your body to continue doing what it knows it needs to do without any conscious interference, overthinking or analysing. This is because the conscious part of the mind is focusing away, with the help of the breath and a vivid yet simple image – a visualisation in your mind.

There are many types of imagery you can visualise when doing the surge breathing. During this part of your course, you will be given the opportunity to practise this effective breathing technique in conjunction with a few different visualisations.

You'll now know that the technique itself is the same regardless of which visualisation you use.

I decided to include this in the book so that you can follow it fully again at home.

The technique starts by taking a slow breath in, through your nose, whilst you count upwards from One. There is no magic number that you need to reach. Just make sure to count slowly because I really believe that if you can slow your counting right down, that will set the pace for slower, more relaxing breaths.

Then, when you have breathed in as much as you can without the need to hold your breath, exhale by allowing the breath to slowly escape through a paper-thin gap between your lips, as you count back down from whichever number you reached on the inward breath. It's absolutely fine if you are still exhaling when you get to zero. Allow that breath to complete entirely before taking the next breath in.

When we exhale, our muscles relax. It is also during the exhalations that we release oxytocin.

'The purpose of surge breathing is to use absolutely the minimum of muscular effort so that the muscles used during the breathing technique do not impact the power of your uterine muscle layers.' – Katharine Graves

The exhalation is not forced at all. Breathing is the easiest way to help us to relax and changing your breath to calm you is within your own power. Think of it as if you are a scuba-diver – the longer the oxygen in the tank on your back lasts, the longer you get to stay underwater. Conserve your breath by slowing it down and you will conserve your energy and your strong birthing resources, helping you to stay calm throughout the duration of your labour and birth.

Slowing down your breath is calming.

Focusing on your breath is calming.

'Breathing is the easiest way to help you to relax.' - The Wise Hippo Birthing Programme

If you'd like to now, why not take a few surge breaths as described above, before allowing your breathing to return to your usual pace and reading on when you are ready.

The balloon visualisation:

The original hypnobirthing (Mongan Method) surge breathing visualisation is of a balloon, and it has been tried and tested since 1989 when the late Marie Mongan founded Hypnobirthing. I practised this technique daily from the moment it was taught to me until my labour started and I then used it continuously for every surge throughout my labour until I was almost fully dilated.

As you inhale through your nose, with your eyes closed, imagine, in your mind's eye, that your breath is filling a big balloon with air and whatever colour you want it to be. The expanding balloon is just above your forehead.

When you have breathed in as much as you can without the need to hold your breath, as you exhale, let the breath slowly escape and watch as your inflated balloon drifts up and away from you in a bright, blue sky. Your balloon appears to be getting smaller and smaller as it floats further and further up and away. At the end of that breath, your balloon disappears beyond the horizon.

If you are still experiencing a surge at that point, with your next slow surge breath, visualise a new balloon in exactly the same way.

You will likely visualise approximately 2 to 5 surge breath balloons during each of your surges.

If you struggle to imagine a balloon inflating as you breathe in, it's possible that you are being very literal about the way you are trying to envisage it because perhaps you think that it is only possible to 'literally' blow up a balloon by exhaling breath out of your mouth into the balloon. What I will say about this is that your mind will visualise what you allow it to. However, a way around this is to picture, as you inhale in through your nose, that you are inflating your belly and that your belly is the balloon. Then, as you let go of the breath, watch your balloon floating up and away in a beautiful, blue sky.

Between the surges, you may like to return to the rest time breathing to conserve your energy and to remain relaxed without any interference from your conscious mind during your rest times.

It can be really helpful to notice how many balloons there are in each surge. This is a reassuring way to measure your surges (not to be confused with timing them). For example, if you have noticed visualising three balloons during each surge, each time you imagine the third balloon expanding, you'll know that very soon the surge will have finished - when you exhale and watch the balloon float away in the bluest of skies - as you let it go, you can feel assured that you are another surge closer to the time when you get to meet, hold and see your baby.

The wave visualisation:

As I live by the sea, I always say to my local clients how very lucky we are to be able to access the beach easily and bring inspiration to our surge breathing by watching the waves as we practice sometimes.

As with the vivid balloon imagery, there are also two ways to visualise the waves when you are breathing through your surges. The first of these is to imagine that you are standing on the beach some way from the shoreline and as you slowly inhale in, you picture in your mind's eye, a wave coming towards the shore. On the exhalation, watch as that wave goes back out to sea. As with the balloon, you will probably start to notice how many surge breaths and waves you experience with each of your surges.

The other way to make use of thinking about a wave during your surges, is to imagine that the wave is all-encompassing of your body and of the sensations you feel. By doing it this way, it is possible to coincide the intensity of the wave in unison with how gentle or powerful your surges feels at any particular time during labour. To breathe & visualise the wave in this way, place your awareness at the tips of your toes at the end of your outward breath. And now draw the breath back in and as you do, imagine that, together with your breath, you are slowly bringing the wave up through your feet, legs, tummy, chest and as far up as you want. On the outward breath, imagine the wave gradually rolling back down over or through your body, legs, feet and away from you, out to the sea and horizon beyond. Picture your exhalation pushing the wave into the distance.

> Practise a few surge breaths every day whilst imagining your chosen visualisation simultaneously (bedtime works well for this - just before playing your Aurora Relaxation for Birth MP3).
>
> Use surge breathing from the very beginning of labour even if you feel like you don't need to.

It is very beneficial to start using the surge-breathing as soon as you feel the first surges of your labour even if you think you don't need a particular breathing technique just yet and could carry on without for a while. This is helpful as it gives you the opportunity to get into the rhythm of each surge and learning how the strongest part of the surge feels. Each surge usually becomes progressively more powerful, reaches a peak before becoming progressively milder until it dissipates. At that point, a rest time will follow until the start of the next surge. If labour is medically monitored, each surge would appear on a graph as a curve, up to the peak and then back down to the end. The rest time would be indicated by a horizontal line until the next surge rises into a peak and then follows a line back down. It can be very useful to get into a breathing pattern with the early surges in such a way that you get used to how the sensation feels for you just before the peak of the surge. If you inhale just before that feeling, this will result in you exhaling through the peak of the surge. This prepares and equips you in advance of more intense surges that might come later as labour progresses.

By exhaling at the peak of a surge, you are going to reduce how strongly the sensation feels during that time. The uterus will still be working just as powerfully and yet the way in which each of those powerful peaks is experienced, will be as though it has plateaued.

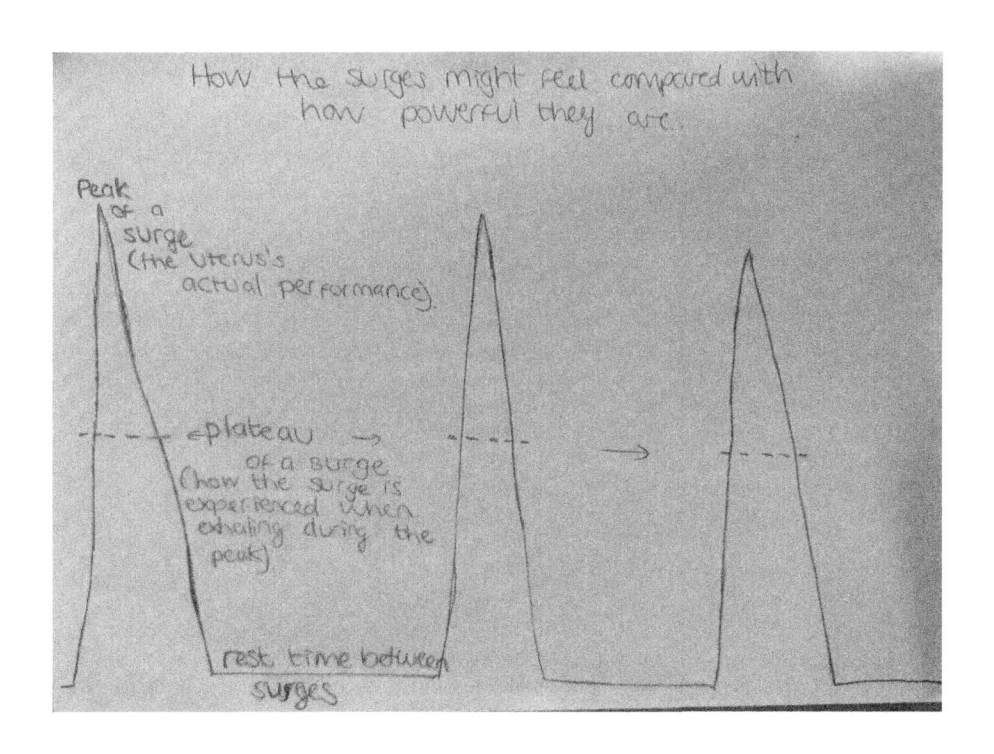

How the surges might feel compared with how powerful they are.

Peak of a surge (the uterus's actual performance)

plateau of a surge (how the surge is experienced when exhaling during the peak)

rest time between surges

Homework:

- Continue to enjoy falling asleep to your MP3s each night.
- If you haven't already done so, read hours 3 to 6 in this book.
- Practise soothing strokes with your partner.
- Practise the birth companion's script at least once before your next class.
- Now that you have learnt Surge Breathing, take two or three surge breaths just before playing Aurora Relaxation for Birth MP3 at bedtime. This will ensure that you are practising surge breathing once a day, every day.
- A nice birth preparation, bedtime routine to do if you have the opportunity with your partner:
    - Enjoy some soft soothing strokes for however long you like whilst practising surge breathing,
    - Practise the birth companion's script without reorientation
    - and then you (or your partner if you've already entered a trance or sleep state) can press play on the bedtime MP3.

In doing this bedtime routine, you are covering lots of techniques in a very short time.

By learning about birth and practising my relaxation techniques, I get to create a calm, empowered internal environment and inner voice on the lead up to and during the time when my baby is born.

HOUR SEVEN

You are now halfway through the material on this course. Well done! I hope you are finding the techniques very relaxing and are feeling confident in your body's ability to do as it needs to when you go into labour and have faith in your capability to birth calmly.

The umbilical cord

Immediately after your baby is born, unless he or she needs urgent medical attention, consider waiting at least until the umbilical cord has stopped pulsating before cutting it. When the cord is pulsating, that means there is still oxygenated blood transferring from the placenta through the cord to the baby. When the baby is born, there is approximately one-third of their volume of oxygenated blood still in the placenta. If you have had a non-water birth or immediately get out of the birth pool after giving birth, about 50% of that remaining oxygenated blood will have transfused through from the placenta to the baby within one minute. After three minutes, about 90% will have been transfused and approximately five minutes after your baby is born, your baby will have received all of his or her oxygenated blood. It's a quick process once the cord has come into contact with the oxygen in the air. However, if you remain in the pool immediately after a water birth, because the umbilical cord will be in water of the same temperature as the amniotic fluid in your uterus, the cord will pulsate more slowly. It can therefore take 20 or 30 minutes for the cord to finish doing its job when you stay in the birth pool. If the midwives mention a concern that could indicate a need to separate mum and baby quite soon after birth, it's worth considering getting out of the water to allow the cord to do its job more quickly.

The placenta

Another benefit of waiting for the umbilical cord to do its job before cutting it, is that by doing so, the volume of the placenta becomes smaller ahead of the third stage.

You can choose whether to have a syntocinon injection (synthetic oxytocin) in your thigh to assist the placenta in detaching from the lining of the womb (active management) or to have a natural third stage. It can take up to an hour for the placenta to come away from the lining of the womb. A midwife or doctor may suggest an assisted third stage if, for example, suddenly a lot of blood is lost as this can be a sign that part of the placenta is retaining. Some women will wait for the third stage to occur naturally and if nothing is happening after a length of time that they are happy waiting for, they will opt for the injection at that stage. It's also good to know that a medically managed third stage does not affect prolactin levels and so is not a concern when thinking about breastfeeding. It can however cause a woman to feel or be sick.

Of course, at that time you will be enjoying those precious first bonding moments with your baby. The midwives will be looking after you and keeping an eye out for any signs that the placenta is on its way or if there are any indications that assistance might be needed.

The placenta, oxytocin and your breast milk

- The presence of the placenta during pregnancy causes high progesterone levels which hinders milk production.
- When your baby and placenta separate shortly after birth, your progesterone drops which triggers the process of milk production.
- Skin-to-skin with your baby and early suckling spikes oxytocin and prolactin release which is a signal to your body to make milk.
- Furthermore, the release of oxytocin makes the alveoli (breast tissue) contract and squeeze the milk through

your breast to your baby.

Skin-to-skin

If you and your baby do need to be separated for any reason, it is great if your birth partner can stay with the baby – even better if this is the baby's other parent. Babies will instinctively be looking for the people they know when they are first born. They will already know their parents' voices and how they smell. In most cases both parents will be with the baby in that early 'golden hour' but if the mother does need urgent attention immediately following the birth, think about whether the partner will go with her or stay with the baby. Newborn babies don't know how long their familiar humans will be gone for and will instinctively bond with who they are given the chance to bond with.

Holding your baby for skin-to-skin is good for so many reasons:

- 'Newborns that have skin-to-skin immediately after birth are more likely to breastfeed within the first hour of their lives. The skin-to-skin contact promotes the release of prolactin for the new mother which is responsible for maintaining breastmilk production.
- Another benefit is that when the baby is placed on his or her mother's chest, the upper part of her body will automatically adjust in temperature according to the climate and how warm or cold the baby is at any given time. Isn't that just wonderful! This way mum and baby regulate the baby's temperature together which is great as babies are otherwise at risk of losing their body heat quickly because they don't have the ability as newborns to shiver in order to keep warm or to pull blankets around them.
- So, skin-to-skin contact helps to increase the baby's body weight as they are not using as much energy to regulate their body temperature by themselves. Instead, the energy can be used to grow.

- However, as mentioned before, if mum and baby do need to spend any time away from each other in the very early bonding minutes and hours immediately following birth, skin-to-skin with the other parent is also beneficial. Both parents will enjoy the emotional benefits and intimacy of skin-to-skin with their baby and knowing that it is also incredibly good for their baby's health and also feels good for the baby.
- Skin-to-skin contact also assists in stabilising the baby's heart rate and calming their breathing patterns. According to Sanford Health, this fabulous work of nature eliminates 75% of heart and breathing issues in newborns.'
- Also from Sanford Health: 'The stress hormone Cortisol is measurably lower after only 20 minutes of skin-to-skin contact. When cortisol and somatostatin are reduced, gastrointestinal problems lessen because it allows for better absorption and digestion of nutrients. When these hormones are reduced, your baby's body can better preserve healthy fat that help maintain their birth weight and keep their body temperature warm.
- Skin-to-skin contact also increases baby's skin hydration, providing a protective barrier that prevents harmful bacteria from entering through baby's skin.
- A new mother's mature immune system passes antibodies through the skin and breast milk to baby.
- During skin-to-skin contact, most infants fall asleep easily and achieve deep sleep, also known as quiet sleep, for an hour or more. Quiet sleep is beneficial for accelerating brain patterning and maturation. Development of mature brain

function in infants is impacted by the quality of a baby's sleep cycle.
- Brain development begins with positive sensory stimulation at birth. Sensations that tell the baby's brain that the outside world is safe include mother's smell, movements and skin-to-skin contact. If the brain does not receive those assurances, brain development does not progress as efficiently. Brain maturation effects are long-term. A study of premature infants showed they had better brain functioning as teenagers compared to adolescents who had been placed in incubators. Researchers attributed it to stabilizing heart rate, oxygenation and improving sleep, which supports the brain to better develop. Another study showed that children who grew up lacking attachment to their parents did more poorly in school and were more likely to be depressed than children who had secure parental attachments. Skin-to-skin contact is one of the earliest steps in forming attachment to parents.'

So, now you know it's good for your baby and why! But did you know that those first snuggles with your baby are also very beneficial to you as well? Here's why:

- When mum and baby are together, hormones that regulate lactation balance out, helping mum to produce more milk and breastfeed more successfully. Newborns' heightened sense of smell helps them seek out the nipple and begin breastfeeding more quickly when placed skin-to-skin. One study showed that mums who practised kangaroo care were more likely to breastfeed exclusively and for longer periods. And mums who were having breastfeeding difficulties saw improvements almost immediately when they started skin-to-skin care one to two times a day for about an hour each time.

- When you are holding your baby skin-to-skin, your oxytocin levels increase, which reduces your blood pressure and lowers stress levels. Increased oxytocin also helps restore pre-pregnancy hormone levels, reducing the risk of postpartum depression.'

(Thank you to Jo Lyn Seitz for her very informative 2017 article written for the Sanford website).

I give myself permission to surrender to the power of my birthing body!

Vitamin K

What is it and what choices do I have for my baby?

We all make Vitamin K in our bodies. In the same way that we convert orange juice into Vitamin C, when we eat avocado, broccoli, blackberries, bacon, cabbage, parsley, etc, etc... a part of that is converted into Vitamin K. Kale is the food containing the highest amount of Vitamin K at 6 times the recommended daily amount. If you have issues with blood clotting or are taking a blood thinning medication such as Warfarin, be wary of this. Please talk to your midwife or doctor if you have any concerns. They will likely suggest a blood test to check your INR (international normalised ratio) reading.

The amount of Vitamin K we have in our body, will determine how quickly our blood congeals. If, for example, we get a scratch on our skin and it bleeds, the number of seconds it takes to coagulate is the INR reading.

Since the 1980s, here in the UK (earlier in America), Vitamin K has been administered to newborn babies – this usually occurs about one hour after birth but it can actually happen anytime in the first 6 hours of your baby's life.

Originally, this could only be administered as an injection but over the last 15 years or so, it has also been possible to ask that your baby receive this in oral drop form. You also have the option of declining. Ultimately, the choice as to whether a baby receives a Vitamin K supplement in the early hours following his or her birth, and if so, in which form, is up to the parents. If parents decide that their baby won't have it, they should talk to the midwife about the warning signs of VKDB so they can look out for these.

The background and reasoning why Vitamin K is recommended

by the World Health Organisation:

During early infancy, when babies are fed entirely on milk, they absorb very little Vitamin K in their diet. A very small number of babies suffer from bleeding due to a lack of Vitamin K. This bleeding may be from the nose, mouth or into the brain. When it occurs in the brain it can be fatal.

In the early 1980s, in England, some hospitals started giving Vitamin K only to newborns that were thought to be at higher risk for bleeding.' – cdc.gov (Centers for Disease Control and Prevention).

Also, from cdc.gov, 'Babies without enough Vitamin K cannot form clots to stop bleeding and they can bleed anywhere in their bodies. The bleeding can happen in their brains or other important organs and can happen quickly. It is rare but when it occurs, infants may need blood transfusions and some need surgery.

Thankfully, the risk of Vitamin K Deficiency Bleeding (VKDB) is small – it affects about 1 in 10,000 full-term babies if they do not get extra Vitamin K.

This means that, in the UK every year, 10 to 20 babies could be brain damaged as a result of a bleed in the brain and four to six babies could die, if Vitamin K was not given. This slight risk is eliminated if a baby is given a big enough dose of Vitamin K.

At one time there were concerns that babies who receive the extra Vitamin K by injection might have an increased risk of developing cancer, including leukaemia, later on in childhood. This link was suggested by a medical study in the early 1990s but since then other studies have been carried out which negated this link. In 1997, a joint expert group of the Medicines Control Agency (MCA), the Committee on Safety of Medicines (CSM) and the Department of Health, considered all these studies. They concluded that, overall, the available data does not support an increased risk of cancer, including leukaemia caused by Vitamin K.

If the Vitamin K supplement is given by mouth, it will need to be repeated at least twice for formula-fed, and three times for breastfed babies over the first month of life in order to be as effective as the injection dose.

Pros and cons for each option:

Declining: Birth is an overwhelming experience for the baby – he or she has never before been cold, hungry, blinded by light, felt the touch of a cloth or the pull of gravity. Some believe that if a baby has had a calm, unassisted vaginal birth (by this I mean that no contact has been made directly with the baby's skull with forceps, ventouse, other tools or a surgeon's hands during crowning), the risk of brain haemorrhage reduces to practically zero. Others will say that surely a mother's body provides everything her unique baby requires during the gestational period and that therefore only babies born prematurely (before 37 weeks gestation) will require a Vitamin K supplement.

Injection: It's over and done with and you know your baby is protected.

Drops: Less discomfort for the baby. The liquid tastes bitter but the taste soon goes away. Offering your baby a feed immediately after giving them a Vitamin K drop, can help whereas a sensation at the site of the injection could last longer. If the baby vomits, a replacement drop will need to be administered. The vial does contain sufficient in case this happens. Also, because the dose administered in injection form is much bigger, drop doses are spread over the first month of the baby's life. This is an additional task to remember during those early weeks with your baby.

When I am
calm and
comfortable
during pregnancy
and birth,
my baby is
calm and
comfortable too.

HOUR EIGHT

Due Dates

One of the first things a lot of women do when they find out they're pregnant is to work out their baby's *estimated due date.* I remember seeing a 'due date calculator wheel' in the surgery waiting room at my booking-in appointment about a week after I had got my positive home pregnancy test. At the time, I thought how good it was to be able to find out with such ease when my baby was due.

Of course, these calculator wheels are only an approximation.

This date is arrived at, assuming that, all women have a 28-day menstrual cycle (which they don't) and ovulate on day 14 (which they don't). Surely it can be said that women with a shorter cycle would probably have a shorter gestational period and someone with a longer cycle will probably have a longer pregnancy. Also, even if a woman does experience 28-day cycles, everyone is unique, and her ovulation might not be on day 14 either.

Furthermore, sperm can survive for up to five days within the female reproductive tract, making fertilisation possible up to five days after sex.

Something else to think about: In Japan, Kenya, France and other countries, a baby's estimated due date is worked out by using a different cycle – the lunar cycle.

It makes a lot of sense, when you think how the tide is pulled in and out to and from the shore and vastly affected by the moon. So many natural events and people's emotions are impacted heavily by the moon's cycle because the human body's composition includes between 45 and 75 per cent of water.

There are more births around or just after a full moon.

Consider taking a look at when the full moon is meant to be happening either side of your 'due date'.

That said, 5% of babies are born on their 'estimated due date' – I was one of them – but this of course means that 95% of them are not.

Your due date is estimated, and a woman is not 'overdue' in her pregnancy (in the UK that is) until she is 42 weeks pregnant. Unless there is a medical indication telling you otherwise, anything from the day you turn 37 weeks until 42 weeks is your due time. I also have my own theory that for women with longer menstrual cycles, perhaps her due time needs to be calculated differently.

In countries where the due time is worked out based on the lunar cycle, a pregnant woman is not post-date until 43 weeks.

Of course, in some cases medical indications give good cause to consider a medicalised induction of labour. However, sometimes further checks can be carried out instead, in many cases, avoiding induction. A bit later in this chapter, I talk about how to ask questions in a way which gains the respect of those supporting you. This helps you to direct the course of your birth.

However, before that, here is a poem reiterating in a beautifully written way, that your baby does not know the due date you have been told. He or she instinctively knows when it's time for them to be born.

A lovely poem called 'We're just fine' to read if you go over your 'due' date:

My baby's not a library book,
so he/she's not overdue.
My baby doesn't over-cook,
coz he/she's not veggie stew.
My baby's not an elephant,
and I'm not fit to burst.
The time and date aren't relevant,
we're blessed with days, not cursed.
My baby can't read dates as yet,
because he/she's very new.
So there's no cause to fuss and fret,
if he/she don't come on cue.
So stop your worry,
stop your asking,
there's no hurry
we're relaxing
in this golden pregnant time,
this pause, which is just his/hers and mine.
You leave us be, we are just fine.

By Rachel Pritchard.

Unless there is a medical reason to induce labour artificially, then usually any advice to do so is merely a suggestion. In the absence of a true medical indication, you may want to consider letting nature take its course.

Here is a list of some of the more natural ways to encourage your baby that it is time for him or her to consider getting ready to be born and to help your body prepare and feel more relaxed about that too (from 37 weeks unless otherwise stated below):

- Arrange a date night with your partner for your estimated due date to focus your energy away from any thoughts or pressure on that particular day.
- Soft soothing strokes on your back and other areas.
- Evening Primrose Oil can be taken in capsule form from 36 weeks.
- Eat hot and spicy foods – but only if you are used to it. If you're used to a Korma, having a Vindaloo may start labour but it could upset your tummy and baby's tummy.
- Scalini's recipe – have a look at their website too (www.scalinis.com) and read stories about mums who ate this meal the day before their babies were born. Scalini's gives pregnant women a voucher to use for another portion of the Eggplant Parmesan if they do not go into labour within 48 hours of eating the meal. If you're local to me, Barolo's in Wimborne Rd, Winton, Bournemouth has also been serving this meal for about 10 years. Take the recipe sheet with you. Or you could prepare the meal with your partner. If my method has reached far and wide since this book was went to print and you are nowhere near Bournemouth, ask your Rose Method Hypnobirthing practitioner if there is a restaurant local to you that is now serving this dish. However you decide to use this idea, bon appetit!
- Intimacy – Kissing, hugging, snuggling up on the sofa,

nipple / clitoral stimulation and sex. All of those things, when enjoyed, will encourage the release of oxytocin. Sex will also help to soften the cervix (it's the prostaglandin in the sperm which does that).

- Eating pineapple – I've heard that the pineapple must be fresh (not tinned) and that it takes the eating of three whole fruits (yes, that includes the core) in one day for it to have the desired effect. Apparently, it's the bromelain in the pineapple that does the trick (prostaglandin has the same ingredient which is why it softens the cervix).

- Acupressure – Apply firm pressure onto the webbed area between your thumb and forefinger on either hand from 37 weeks. I believe this works as it releases tension. It is also the pressure point for relieving tension headaches.

- Acupuncture – Very effective. Mark Arnold of Bournemouth Acupuncture (www.bournemouthandpoole-acupuncture.co.uk) has his main clinic in Redhill where he works on a Monday, Tuesday and Wednesday and he works from his Broadstone clinic on Thursdays and Fridays. Abbey at Eclipse in Luther Road (www.eclipse-acupuncture.co.uk) is also great. I have used Mark and Abbey myself and highly recommend them. I've heard good things about Rachel Dufft in Southbourne and also Jill Booth in Bournemouth too. If my method has reached far and wide since this book was went to print and you are nowhere near Bournemouth, ask your Rose Method Hypnobirthing practitioner if there is someone she can recommend.

- Reflexology – Some reflexologists refuse to use their techniques to induce labour because they know how powerful it is and don't want to interfere with the natural process of body and baby doing their thing. However, many others think that reflexology is a gentler method of encouraging labour to start than using synthetic hormones. I tend to agree. Locally, here in Bournemouth, I recommend Lisa Wijsveld (soul2solebournemouth.wordpress.com). She is fantastic at what she does and I have been recommending her for many years with excellent feedback from clients. If you also live within a reasonable radius of Lisa, I can't recommend her highly enough. She is a mobile reflexologist too and will travel to you for labour-inducing reflexology. Simonne of Bournemouth Reflexology (www.bournemouthreflexology.co.uk) is also excellent. If you are in a different location, your Hypnobirthing practitioner will hopefully be able to recommend someone near you.

- Laughing / crying – Both of these release tension and I highly recommend watching some stand-up comedy or a funny / emotional film. At the same time, you could use the acupressure technique and snuggle on the sofa with your partner, your older child, or your pet.
- Play your Aurora Relaxation for Birth, Words of Conscious Reaffirmation or Emotional Clearing MP3. This is especially effective if you fall asleep as you're more likely to go into labour when you are as relaxed as possible and you can't really get a more relaxed state than sleep.
- Have a warm, relaxing bath.
- Go for a walk.
- Use your 'BRAINS' – remember, in the absence of a true medical indication, it's safe to let labour start spontaneously instead of being medically induced. You may be asked to go into hospital for monitoring every other day but on one of those days, it's very likely that you won't need to go in to be monitored as labour will have started on its own.

The BRAINS' questions are good to ask if you are in an appointment with a midwife or consultant doctor during your pregnancy and something is being suggested in what might feel like a routine way, despite you knowing nothing or very little about what it entails. This can also be used during your labour when your partner will be your spokesperson during that time.

B: BENEFITS - What are the BENEFITS of what is being suggested?

R: REASONS and RISKS – What REASONS are being put forward by the person proposing the intervention. For example, in the case of scheduling an induction for a date in the future, 'What REASON do you see right now, that it indicates to you, that I need to have my baby on that date?' What are the RISKS of what's being suggested? How might it impact the rest of my labour and birth?

A: ALTERNATIVES – What are the ALTERNATIVES of what is being suggested? An example might be monitoring the baby's movements straightaway if the concern is that these have reduced. If such monitoring ascertains that everything is fine with you and everything is fine with the baby and that was the only reason given, it is unlikely that you would need to have your labour induced. Of course, it is your choice.

I: your INSTINCTS and IMPACT on you – How do you feel about what is being suggested. Listen to your gut intuition. How does it make you feel when you consider what is being suggested?

N: is it NECESSARY right NOW? For example, 'Is it NECESSARY right NOW that we schedule an induction in our diaries for a certain date? I would prefer to review things on that date please.' In the absence of a current medical indication right NOW, a medical intervention is not a requirement. It can also feel like a race against the clock to be told you will be induced on a certain date if you haven't gone into labour spontaneously before then. And that feeling can cause worry in the mind which in turn can cause tension in the body which can prevent labour from starting on its own. And all of that can be avoided by declining something if it is not NECESSARY in the exact moment it is being discussed or suggested.

S: say it with a SMILE. Nobody wants to appear challenging towards the midwives and doctors who have their health and the health of their baby in mind as they discuss options. A conversation can be assertive and kind. It can be a friendly chat in which you explain that you want to make the right choice for you and your baby and that you are really grateful for all the information being shared to help you do that.

The main thing to remember, when asking any BRAINS questions, is that you are discussing your body, your baby and your birth experience. The job of the medical professionals that look after you during your pregnancy, labour, and birth journey, is to support and guide you. They are a mine of information – much of which you will never need to know. However, asking relevant questions if the time comes to make a decision, will better equip and prepare you with the information needed to ensure that choice is a well-informed one and enable YOUR birth experience to be directed by YOU. You are the expert of you at all times, especially in the absence of a medical indication. If certain things take a medical turn, you are still the expert of yourself but take advantage of the people who are there to look after you. Ask them a question. Ask them another question. Ask them more questions. It's perfectly normal and human to be interested or curious about what your body and baby are doing or are about to do.

I also just want to say that I think people make better decisions about things if they are given time to think about the facts they have been told and how they feel. So, once you have asked the questions you want answered, it is highly unlikely that it would be imperative for you to decide there and then what you would like to do. I think a useful phrase might be something along the lines of, 'Thank you so much for all of the information. There is so much to think about and I really appreciate you sharing your knowledge. I'd like to go home and talk it over with my husband and consider how I feel about what you have recommended.'

- If your waters have broken but surges have not started and quite some time has passed, induction may also be recommended because of the increased risk of infection for your baby. Did you know that the risk of infection is 1 in 200 when the membranes are intact, and this increases to 1 in 100 once your waters

break. In this case, if you wish, you can request antibiotics instead. This is a highly effective way of eliminating the risk of infection which is usually the reason induction is being suggested. If there are other reasons, remember the BRAINS questions.
- Eating 6 dates a day from 36 weeks. This reduces induction and augmentation (speeding up labour). Study in Jordan (https://www.ncbi.nlm.gov/m/pubmed/21280989/)

96% of women who ate 6 dates a day in the 4 weeks leading up to her due date went into labour spontaneously. 79% of the control group did (they ate no dates in that period).

28% of those who consumed dates had syntocinon / pitocin (synthetic oxytocin) administered to augment (speed up) labour. This compared with 47% of the women who ate no dates.

I believe that if you added Hypnobirthing to the equation, the statistics would show even less need for medical intervention (for ALL women – date-eating or not)

- **Ask questions and remember, YOU are always the EXPERT of YOUR BODY. The medical staff are the experts if there is a medical reason.**

Natural uterine tonic:

Raspberry Leaf Tea – Although there is no evidence that this brings on labour, it definitely does tone the uterus. Start drinking this from 36 weeks. You can also buy it in supplement form if you prefer that to the loose tea or teabags.

AVOID:

There is an old wives' tale that says that taking two tablespoons of castor oil will induce labour. It's something which our grandmothers possibly considered doing and I have met a few ladies who have said it worked for them. However, as with the very spicy curries, if you're not used to it, castor oil may upset your tummy and possibly also your baby's tummy. I would therefore advise you to avoid this. I've heard that it tastes foul anyway. A gentler alternative is to add a couple of drops of lavender or clary sage oil to caster oil and to use that to massage your abdomen in a clockwise direction for a few minutes every day.

I trust that my body knows exactly what to do to make, grow and bring my baby to me.

HOUR NINE

Remember that when you're pregnant, your body is working together with your baby to get you both ready for birth. Your body and your baby are instinctively doing everything necessary to reach as optimum a state as possible in time for labour and birth:

Your hormone levels change to help soften your cervix.

Natural lubrication occurs and the birth path smooths out in preparation for your baby's journey to meet you.

By giving yourself time to rest, playing calming music and listening to your Rose Method MP3s, your body relaxes, and this gives your baby the necessary room to naturally adjust to the vertex, head down position in the uterus.

Relaxation creates more room in the womb for your baby.

Other ways in which you can encourage your baby to get and stay in this left occiput anterior (LOA) position – baby on the left side of the uterus, head down, back to belly) :

Sleep on your left side. If your baby adopts an ROA (right occiput anterior) position late on in pregnancy, he or she might instinctively rotate to LOA to be born. To do this, babies move in a clockwise directions with the centrifugal force of nature, resulting in a period of back-to-back labour.

Ensure that you're sitting so that your knees are level with or lower than your hips. This will mean that the front of your uterus is lower than the back of your uterus and the baby's back with gravitate to the lowest side of the uterus. Birth balls are good for this. They usually come in a choice of sizes. 55cm tends to be perfect for anyone up to 5'1", 65cm those between 5'2" & 5'7" and 75cm if you are 5'8" or taller. Double-check the individual manufacturer's guidelines when choosing the right size for you. Ensure you fully inflate the ball.

Regular rest times also help you to release hormones that are conducive to further relaxation, and this inhibits the secretion of stress hormones (aka catecholamines).

Your pelvic structure adjusts to accommodate the specific anatomical makeup of *your* baby and the descent of *your* baby – your body contains your baby's DNA from the moment of conception onwards and so your body knows *exactly* what to do when preparing for your baby's birth. Nature knows.

Your baby's skull has fontanels – soft spots – one at the top and one at the back. Because the fontanels are soft, this allows the parts of the skull to move and overlap like plates. During birth, your baby's head will mould itself to the perfect shape and size to fit through the birth path and for crowning. After your baby is born, the fontanels at the back of the skull fuse solid pretty much straightaway. The ones on the top of the head remain soft and you will notice this area pulsating until your baby is about one year old.

I imagine that my placenta detaches and emerges easily.

The perineum

Here are some things a woman can do to give herself the greatest chance of an intact perineum after birth:

- Perineal massage from 34 weeks (see below).
- Gradual birth breathing instead of forced pushing and straining (see Hour 11).
- A warm compress applied to the perineal area, during the birthing stage, to relax the muscles.
- Avoiding episiotomy without good reason. Episiotomies are more likely than spontaneous tears to result in third- or fourth-degree tears and tearing heals more easily than an episiotomy.
- A standing or squatting position during the birthing stage (squatting also shortens and widens the birth path).
- A water birth.

Perineal massage increases the elasticity in the one area which stretches during childbirth. Your birth path will open to be receptive to your baby's journey, however your perineum will stretch. Imagine how the circumference of an elastic band starts off small but if it is supple and flexible, will easily expand without tearing. Each time you do the perineal massage, you will likely feel a slight sting as you stretch the area. The next time you do it, you will no longer feel a sting when massaging to the exact same point as the previous day. You'll be able to massage a little further before feeling the slight sting. Do this for a few minutes once a day from 34 weeks until labour starts, and you will increase the elasticity day by day.

It's absolutely fine to use olive oil or almond oil that you most probably already have at home but if you want to buy a specially formulated one you can.

There is also a gadget you can buy called an Epi-no which you insert and pump up, and which does the massaging for you, as well as measuring how much you have increased the elasticity by.

Towards the end of this book, I talk about the other major thing that will help you to avoid tearing – it's all in the birth breath. I wish I could guarantee that by doing these things, your perineum will remain intact – I think that's the biggest concern for most women – what I will say is that perineal massage from 34 weeks (or as soon as you are reading this if that's later – every little really does make a difference) either manually or with an Epi-no gadget (done by either you or your partner) increases the perineum's capacity to stretch which thereby removes the need for an episiotomy or tearing in most cases. It also makes for a more comfortable, crowning stage. That's got to be worth a few minutes of your time every day for a few weeks, hasn't it?

One of Weleda's reps and a hypnobirthing client of mine provided amazing pamper treatments using Weleda products at my 2019 Pregnant Pause retreat and she also handed out some Weleda literature which included useful perineal massage information and drawings. I have shared some information below taken from that literature so that you know exactly what to do to prepare and increase the elasticity in your perineum ready for the birth of your baby:

'What and where is the perineum?

The perineum is the small area of firm skin and muscular tissue between the vagina and the anus. The perineum plays a significant role in women's health. This muscular tissue connects with pelvic floor muscles, offering support to the pelvic organs. It works extra hard in pregnancy due to the extra weight it bears. Tearing of the perineum during childbirth can weaken this support, making later pelvic floor problems or prolapse of the uterus more likely. Massaging the perineum helps keep the connective tissues supple and elastic - our best defence against tearing. Massage helps increase the perineum's capacity to stretch more easily and less painfully during birth.

When can I start? Recommended from the 34th week of pregnancy, using a perineum massage oil is a great way to nurture your body and prepare for birth. Massage 3-4 times a week for 5-10 minutes. A good time is after a relaxing bath or warm shower when blood vessels in the area are dilated and this makes the perineum softer and more comfortable to touch.

Do not massage if you have any infection. Empty your bowel and bladder before starting.

Begin by placing both hands on your perineum and just relax about touching this part of your body. We can hold a lot of tension around the perineum, and releasing any tension here is good preparation for birth. Pour a little oil into your hands and rub them together to warm them. Then gently smooth oil over the whole of your perineum. Stroke in whatever way feels comfortable for you. Get to know the different areas of skin - some soft and delicate, and some firm and more muscular which will stretch out in labour. Massage this a little more firmly. You could apply a little pressure here as you breathe out. Try doing your pelvic floor exercises. As you breathe out, draw up your pelvic floor and as you breathe in, relax. Make sure that your buttocks are not tightening. Make the exercises harder by tightening the muscles gradually on your out-breath, imagining that you are going up floors in a lift. Go down the floors with the in-breath. Don't clench your jaw: relaxing your jaw in labour can help relax your perineum. You can also do some gentle pulsing, tightening and releasing, as you breathe out. If you feel comfortable, you can try doing these exercises with a finger or thumb inside your vagina.

In the last few weeks of pregnancy, you can try stretching out the perineum to prepare for birth. To do this, place your finger or thumb inside your vagina up to the second knuckle, and gently massage in a rhythmic U-shaped movement the lower part of the vaginal opening nearest to the anus (from 3 o'clock to 9 o'clock). This will gently stretch the vaginal tissues and muscles. As you feel comfortable, you can try increasing the pressure and adding in a stretch back towards the anus. This may sting slightly; this stinging sensation occurs for many women when the baby's head is born.'

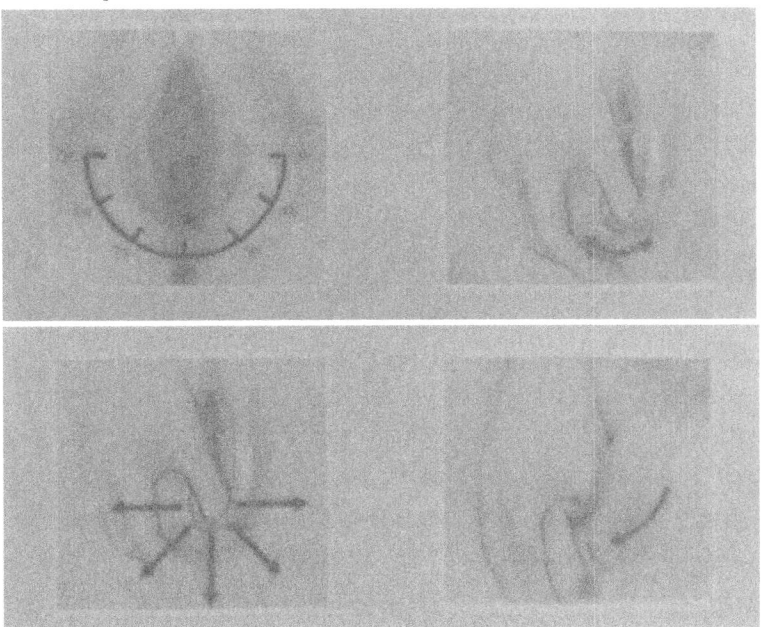

Drawings are from Weleda's pregnancy brochure.

I was fortunate to chat to Teresa of Epi-No whilst I was writing this section of the book. Teresa shared some very interesting information about the benefits of using an Epi-No, clinical trial results and how using one differs from perineal massage without a device.

The Epi-No is a great option for women who feel unsure if they are doing the perineal massage effectively.

The great thing about the Epi-No is that it tracks the progress you make each time you use it so that you know how much you have increased the elasticity of your perineum after each 'stretch'. I learnt, when talking with Teresa, that it involves inflating a balloon part of the device inside the vagina – the amount by which you inflate it, increases gradually day by day.

EPI-NO STATISTICS.

Following clinical trials, compared with the control group who did not use an Epi-No or even do any manual perineal massage, 48% of the ladies who got their perineum ready by increasing the elasticity by using the Epi-No, had an intact perineum after giving birth. 8.5% of the control group did.

78% of the women in the control group had an episiotomy (where a medical professional makes a surgical incision during the second stage {just before the baby is born} to give the baby's head more space to crown) and 42% of those who did their perineal birth training with an Epi-No had an episiotomy.

I believe that it's primarily a combination of perineal massage and the birth breathing which will give you the greatest chance of having an intact perineum (no tearing or episiotomy) during crowning. The mindset and trust a woman has in her own body and in the birth process, that comes from attending a hypnobirthing course and practising at home, is a huge factor that will make an enormous difference to the outcome of using this combination of effective techniques.

'Perineal massage can also help tone the muscles after birth. Start gentle massage as soon as you feel comfortable.'

I stop unnecessary interference by relaxing my conscious mind.

HOUR 10

How do you feel about labour and birth now that you are equipped with a toolbox full of techniques to practise using and to take with you into your birth experience? Have your mindset and expectations changed in any way? Do you feel better prepared than you did at the start of your hypnobirthing journey?

Imagine that we have gone forward in time to the moment when your baby is ready to be born and you notice those first surges of labour. What do you think you will do? How will you feel? Will those factors depend on the time of day or night? Lots of labours start when a woman is sleeping as that is when we are feeling most relaxed and feeling relaxed is conducive to telling the body that it is ready and not busy dealing with other things / worrying / in survival or fight or flight mode.

Have a think about how you can make both your external environment (the people, things, sounds, smells, etc you are surrounding yourself with) and your internal environment (your mind) conducive to relaxation so that your nervous system knows it's ok to relax right now. See Hours 4 and 5 in this book again to recap on ways in which you can make positive changes to your external and internal environment.

When we feel safe and relaxed, we release an amazing cocktail of hormones which tell us, once the time's right, that we're ready to go into labour.

The first of those hormones is oxytocin – I love that this literally means Oxygenated Birth. Breathing in a calm way increases the amount of oxygen flowing through your body and that in itself helps birth to happen.

Oxytocin is your calm birth fuel and if you let it, it will flow in abundance.

It might seem too obvious to even mention, however, the easiest way we can help ourselves relax is through the way that we breathe.

During the first surges, it might feel like you are absolutely fine carrying on with your day without doing anything any differently and that you don't need to start any special breathing techniques yet.

Do it anyway!

Using the surge breathing that you have learnt and have been practising since around your second hypnobirthing session, from the very start of your labour, will help you for many reasons:

- This is your first opportunity to use surge breathing with actual surges.
- Getting into a rhythm and noticing where the peak of the surge is and how that feels, will really help. When using surge breathing and exhaling through the peak or most intense part of a surge, your uterus will be working very powerfully doing exactly what it needs to – however, the way you experience that surge will be quite different. By starting to use the surge breathing together with your chosen visualisation as soon as labour starts, no matter how gentle those early surges feel, you will have the opportunity to notice when the intensity of the surge increases. This way, you can feel into the sensations and inhale just ahead of the peak of the surge. In doing this, you will be exhaling through the most intense part of the surge, enabling the surge

to plateau. It will feel as though your exhalation has cut off the peak.
- It is on the outward breaths during labour that we release oxytocin. Exhalations during surge breathing are thereby signalling the release of oxytocin for a greater amount of time than would be the case when taking shallow breaths.
- All of our other muscles relax when we exhale, enabling the uterus to work more efficiently without other muscle groups in the body pulling resources from it.
- Functions of the human body are more comfortable when we let go of our breath rather than hold it.
- By breathing and visualising you are using the creative part of your mind and helping yourself to shut out any unnecessary thoughts and questions by focusing away from any conscious interference. In Hour 11, I talk about what a huge difference this can make to the moment of transition.
- A surge builds up to a peak and then becomes less intense before it completes. Breathing through your surge will help to keep you calm through that time.
- Another thing some of my clients have found useful is to measure the length of the surges with their breath. This is made possible through the imagery you create in your mind. This is not the same as timing them. You do not need to be concerned with how much time is passing or what time it is as doing so can cause conscious thinking interference. When you have been in labour for a while you might start to notice some regularity to your surges. It may become apparent, for example, that each surge is three balloon visualisations or three wave visualisations long (three surge breaths). This can be very helpful

and motivating. Imagine that is the case for you, so that when you reach the third time during a surge, of picturing your wave rolling into the shore or your balloon filling with air and whatever colour you choose for it to be, you can be almost certain that at the end of this very breath, your surge will be over and you will have some rest time. This is possible by noticing a consistent surge pattern or rhythm and it really does help lots of women when they utilise their surge-breathing visualisations in that way.

Your body will have a rest times between your surges, during which you can enjoy some Esdaille resting breaths until the next surge begins.

As mentioned in Hour Six, I hope your birth partner will take responsibility for timing the gaps between the surges until you travel to the birth centre or hospital or, if you're planning a home birth, until your midwife arrives with you.

Signs for your birth partner to look out for when starting to time the gaps between your surges (from the end of one surge until the beginning of the next one):

- During a surge your eyes will probably be closed or dreamy looking, especially when you are taking advantage of the surge breathing already – something I highly recommend you doing.
- The rise and fall of the chest will be noticeably different during surge breathing than during those rest times between them.
- The uterus will rise and stay risen during a surge.

The Purple Line

Another thing your partner can look for is the purple vertical line on your lower back. This appears in labour and becomes longer as your cervix dilates.

The purple line appearance in the expectation of labour progress had 85.25% accuracy – Sara Wickham.

The purple line was more likely to be seen in women experiencing spontaneous labour than in those whose labours had been induced – Farrag et al (2021)

The purple line is sometimes quite faint and sometimes quite bold and it is present in about 90% of labours.

Checking for dilation via the purple line method is less invasive and places less risk of infection on the baby than vaginal examinations does.

The line will start at your anus and rise upwards and its length in correlation to cervical dilation can vary by a centimetre or so between individuals.

www.wildwoodbirth.pdx.com/purple-line-dilation
is an excellent resource with real images of the purple line.

Purple Line Length	Estimated Cervix Dilation
3-6cm	1-2cm
5-8cm	3-6cm
7-9cm	7-8cm
8-11cm	9-10cm

(Figures take from wildwoodbirth.pdx.com)

My body is making way, perfectly, for my baby's journey.

As well as starting to use the surge-breathing together with your preferred visualisation from the start of labour, you may also like to think about other tangible anchors for your home (see Hour Four and Five for a recap on these). This is certainly the case if you are planning for a home birth but it's also useful if you want a hospital birth, as your home will likely be your environment until surges are approximately 3 to 5 minutes apart – the time you leave for the birth centre will depend how long a journey you have to reach it, whether it is rush hour or the middle of the night, etc… Listen to your body and go to the hospital earlier if you have any concerns – always trust your gut instinct on this.

If you are planning a home birth, you may have already agreed that your partner will phone the home birth team when labour starts and will keep them updated on progress. They may also give them another call when your surges are 3 to 5 minutes apart. It's possible your midwife may pop in and see you before that if you would like them to. The good thing about this is that they will come and go whilst you remain in the comfort of your chosen birth environment.

If you are opting to give birth in a hospital or birth centre, when you feel it is time to make your journey there, it's a good idea for your partner to call them and let them know.

Questions that the hospital staff will likely ask your partner during that phone call:

'How is your partner responding to the labour?'

'Do you know how far apart the surges are?'

They may also ask to speak to you. I don't think this is of benefit to anyone. You may be perfectly able to speak during a surge because you are feeling very calm. However, that depth of calm could be affected if you start to have an unnecessary conversation. Your partner can simply explain that you are doing Hypnobirthing. The midwives are sometimes listening to a labouring woman's voice for signs that she is in established labour. One reason for this is to dissuade people from going in too soon. However, it is very common for Hypnobirthing women to sound very calm throughout labour – during surges and between them. So, this conversation could be misleading for the midwives in any case. You may be capable of speaking during your surges, however do you want to?

Your partner can then also ask questions on your behalf. Here are a few ideas:

'Do you have a midwife on duty who has supported a lot of hypnobirths recently? If so, please could we be allocated that midwife?'

Or

'Is our regular midwife on duty at the hospital today? We'd like them to be a part of our birth if that's possible.'

If you are hoping to have a water birth, it's a good idea for your partner to ask on the phone about having a room with a birth pool and if they could start filling the pool. That way, whilst you are making your way there, they can start getting this ready for you.

Maybe you could spend a little time, together with your partner, making a short list of questions for them to remember to ask during that phone call and they could save this as a memo on their phone. Also get them to add the hospital's phone number to their contacts.

My uterus relaxes between surges to give my baby the time and space needed to move down.

Making your way to the hospital / birth centre

If you are planning to have your baby in a hospital or a birth centre, there are things you can do to help make your journey there as calm and comfortable as possible.

During all other times (at home and in the birth centre / hospital or any other labouring and birthing environment you have chosen), it's great to listen to your music or MP3s through your headphones – that way you are less likely to get interrupted or pulled out of your deeply relaxed state if there are any noisy conversations going on around you. However, I'd recommend also playing it through a speaker, so that anyone else in the room can hear it too. If the midwives have the radio blaring, they are likely to be in a different headspace. If everyone (including your birth partner) is exposed to the same music as you, they'll be on the same page as you and they'll likely also feel calmer and better able to support you.

Also, if you decide to take your headphones / earphones / airpods out for a while, the MP3 or relaxing music will still be playing for you.

However, in the car en route to the birth centre, if listening to your MP3s, this should be played only through headphones whilst the driver, (likely your birth partner), tunes into the radio to stay alert. Remember, they are also likely to have created an associated link between the MP3 and feeling relaxed, especially if they have been falling asleep to it at night since you started your hypnobirthing course.

I had a 20-minute journey between where we lived and the maternity unit in Poole and the position I found most comfortable was to be semi-reclined on my side in the passenger seat. I must have been on my right side because Pete was aware of when I was having a surge by noticing my uterus rise and fall. I think by being reclined, I felt unobserved by anyone outside of the car, despite it being very busy as it was about 9.30am on a Saturday morning. I know it might seem crazy because no one would have had a clue that I was in labour anyway, but it's our own interpretation of being aware that there are people around that is what matters and impacts the psycho-physical responses. Privacy, safety and comfort are super-important.

You might also like to put a blanket over you in the car if it's a cold day or the middle of the night. An eye-mask can also help.

For a small minority of women, labour might speed up during the journey to the hospital. Maybe they'll feel less comfortable at home because they have made a decision that they want to be in a medical environment and so now they're on their way to the place where they feel they will be safe, the body lets go and surrenders to the surges.

For a lot of women, the surges will remain as they were.

And for some women, things will slow down a little, because most women don't want to have their baby in the car.

However this gets to be for you, it's all fine. Remember, the car journey is just a small proportion of your labour. See it as an extended rest time between surges if things do slow down. And if things accelerate, that's ok too.

I trust my body and the process of giving birth.

HOUR 11

Arrival at the hospital / birth centre.

If parking is scarce next to the birth unit as can be the case at Poole, get your partner to pull in next to the front door of the hospital, bring in any bags and leave the car there for a short while until you are allocated a midwife. Your partner can then go and park the car. In Poole, there is a multi-storey car park next to the main hospital which is about a 3-minute walk from the maternity unit. A good idea is to pay for 24 hours if that's an option and then forget about it.

The midwives will likely take you straight into the room they have allocated for you knowing that you were on your way in. They will do their initial checks – for example, checking your baby's heart rate.

Vaginal examinations and other intervention.

On arrival, if you like you can ask the midwife to ascertain how far dilated your cervix is. You may even be offered this. However, it is always up to you to decide if you would like to be examined or not, if you would like any medical pain relief, if you agree to any procedures or not. How could it possibly be anyone else's decision but yours whether someone puts their fingers inside your vagina? Always keep in mind that, even if something sounds like it is being offered to you in a rather routine way, you always have a choice whether you want them to do it or not. It is always absolutely fine and a very good idea, especially if you are undecided about any examinations or interventions, to ask questions before agreeing to them. You are within your right to ask how the intervention being suggested might impact the rest of your labour and birth and what the alternatives, benefits and risks might be. Remember the BRAINS from Hour 8 earlier in this book (Benefits, Risks and Reasons, Alternatives, your Instincts, is it Necessary right Now? and Say it with a Smile).

'Woman must not accept; she must challenge. She must not be awed by that which has been built up around her; she must reverence that woman in her which struggles for expression.' – Margaret Sanger

My body is healthy and grows my baby to a healthy size that I can give birth to.

Transition.

During the first stage of labour, the purpose of the surges is to cause the cervix to open and dilate. The second stage is where the uterus pushes your baby out of your vagina. Between those two stages is transition.

As birthing advances, nature provides an amnesiac state that relaxed labouring women will naturally fall into. This takes a woman deeper into her birthing energy and promotes connection with her baby.

Most of the time when we're awake, we all predominantly use the left side of our brains. That's the thinking, problem-solving, solution-finding, analytical side which we rely on to go about our daily routine and to carry out tasks. Someone who is very creative or has a very creative job (for example an artist, actor, writer etc) will use their feminine, creative, right side a little more than the rest of us do, but even they are using the left side the most.

During labour, and specifically at the point of transition, the right side – that feminine, creative part – takes over completely and this is the mind's way of enabling birth to happen without unnecessary overthinking, worrying, etc... Clients have said to me what a shame it is that this mind-transition doesn't happen at the very start of the dilation phase, when that first surge happens. That would be handy, wouldn't it? Seriously though, there's a reason why the transition of state of mind occurs when it does, or rather there is a reason why your body and mind think they don't require this massive mind-shift during the first stage of labour, and that's because your body and mind are not born with a fear of labour and birth and your body and mind know that you have all of the phenomenal power, coping hormones and ability to do exactly what it is you need to do so that your cervix will dilate and get you to the 'pushing' stage. Your body and mind are 100% right in this knowledge. The issue is that today, in the western world, it is common for people to be conditioned and programmed from a young age that labour and birth are painful, medical and messy. Many are exposed to traumatic images of birth in films and tv programmes – the media has a lot to answer for! I recall being petrified about the idea of getting a baby out of me after watching an apparently 'educational' birth film at school. It had such a profound effect on my psyche for many years even when I'd put it to the back of my mind.

I'd like you to consider something for a moment. How is your experience during the opening phase likely to differ to that of someone who has not attended hypnobirthing classes? What will you be doing throughout that first stage?

When you do those things – the deep breathing and visualising - you are already using the creative side of your brain. Sometimes, when hypnobirthing is being used, the midwives don't notice transition because, by that time, a hypnobirthing woman is so relaxed in her creative right brain headspace that there is little to no mind-shift being experienced.

You're a birthing goddess!

This is such a contrast from the signs that midwives are used to seeing - signs that indicate when a woman is ready for the birth stage. Women who have expressed firmly, all the way through labour until this point, that they do not want to be offered any pain relief, may suddenly request an epidural or Caesarean, and I have heard of cases where the woman has stood up and left the room, looking very confused as to her reason for being there at all (that's the amnesiac effect), only to return minutes later to say that the baby's head is crowning. However, for a woman practising hypnobirthing, this stage often goes unnoticed by the medical staff and even the birthing mother herself.

One of the films I have shown in the past during my classes, is Claire's birth. Claire had a home water birth. When the time came and she felt her baby's head crowning, she said to the midwife (who was still adding warm water to the pool at the time), 'I'm having my baby.' The midwife replied by telling her that she 'had a while to go yet'. Just moments later, Claire exclaimed excitedly, 'I've had my baby!'

The midwife was taken by complete surprise and was left with no time to put a surgical glove on and take her watch off before reaching into the pool to catch and bring baby into Claire's arms.

Claire is a prime example of a woman in her intuitive power, trusting the birth process and also being in her relaxed headspace before the point of transition, meaning that it was very hard for anyone, apart from Claire herself to know that she was close to giving birth. What a birthing goddess!

I breathe as my
uterus rises
and
nudges my baby
down to meet me.

Birth breathing.

During the dilation phase, you can feel your surges, but you cannot directly feel the purpose of them (you cannot tell that your cervix is opening). During the birthing phase, you can feel the impact of the surges as your uterus pushes your baby down to be born. The purpose of birth breathing is not to get your baby out - your powerful longitudinal uterus muscle fibres will do that - but what birth breathing will do is give you somewhere else to channel the energy that might otherwise cause you to want to forcefully strain because of a conditioned urge and belief that we need to exert effort to 'push' our babies out.

So, what is the difference between forced pushing and birth breathing and why on earth am I suggesting that you don't push? Women do push their babies out, right?

Once your cervix is fully dilated to 10cm open, and the baby is ready to move through the birth path you reach the latent phase of the expulsion stage. This is when the uterus takes on the role of nudging your baby down. This active phase is where the purpose of your uterine surges is to push the baby out.

The force of nature can feel overwhelmingly powerful, and it is common to experience an unstoppable urge to somehow 'push' by squeezing and tensing the smooth muscle sphincters. When those sphincters are squeezed and tensed, they will grip the baby's head and propel it along the birth path. However, for this to happen, the woman must hold her breath for the duration of each forced 'push'. Each time she lets go of her held breath, she will simultaneously release the vaginal grip on her baby's head. This causes any forward progression that has been made during the time she's been holding her breath, to be reversed because when we release the tension which is forcing something forward or holding something in place, it will move back.

'For every action there is an equal and opposing reaction.' - Newton's third law of motion.

Newton's Third Law of Motion states that for every action, there is an equal and opposite reaction. What this means is that pushing on an object causes that object to push back against you, the exact same amount, but in the opposite direction.

Here's a little analogy for you: Imagine you are at the end of your toothpaste tube. You know there is just about enough toothpaste left in the tube to brush your teeth this time, so you squeeze the tube really hard, and a little toothpaste can be seen over the rim of the tube. As you go to pick up your toothbrush and release your grip on the tube, the toothpaste immediately goes back into the space where the pressure and tension was applied. This is exactly what happens to a baby's head when his or her mother releases the strained pushing and tension that she was forcefully squeezing her baby down the birth path with.

'A pregnant woman is like a beautiful flowering tree but take care when it comes time for the harvest that you do not shake or bruise the tree, for in doing so you may harm both the tree and its fruit.' – Peter Jackson.

Should a midwife suggest that you push, know that you are pushing.

There is a fine line between feeling as though you are forcefully pushing and the involuntary pushing which your uterus is doing. Of course, it feels like you are pushing because you are. Your uterus is part of you and so of course you are going to feel those expulsive reflex nudges.

The imagery I like and which I have taught everyone on my course to use, is the Mongan Method rose picture. It's been tried and very successfully tested by hypnobirthing women globally since 1989 when hypnobirthing was founded by the late Marie Mongan herself. An opening rose is a beautiful imagery and there are similarities between the process of the cervix dilating during labour, the birth path opening during birth and a flower gradually transforming from bud to full bloom of petals, just as nature intended.

I have also included some affirmation photos of rosehip flowers from my garden which would also work well as a birth breathing visualisation.

Birth breathing is mother-directed breathing where a labouring woman follows the lead of her body. This is possible as long as a woman has not had an epidural. A woman who has had an epidural will be unable to feel the uterus contracting. When a woman has had an epidural, she will be hooked up to a monitor which shows the midwives the progression and intensity of each surge, as a wave on a graph, and the baby's heart rate is also constantly measured alongside this, so that the midwives can see how the baby is responding to the surges.

Birth breathing is an option in all cases – you would need look at the monitor or be told when you are experiencing a surge if you have had an epidural, as you will be unable to feel them.

It is a technique that works, as I said before, by giving you somewhere to focus the energy which might otherwise cause you to feel like forcefully pushing. Forceful pushing or straining causes tension in the birth path which at that time, more than any other, needs to be relaxed and open – the complete opposite of what forced, purple pushing does (so called because many women cause themselves bloodshot eyes and burst capillaries in the skin of their face because of all the unnecessary tension and breath-holding).

Other hypnobirthing methods refer to this birth breathing technique as, J-breathing (because of the j-shape of the breath) and birth humming.

Birth breathing involves a short intake of breath directed in through the nose (the top of the letter 'J') to the back of the throat and then a long exhalation which can be imagined as being channelled down the body (the stem of the 'J). The tail of the 'J' or the opening rose imagery are helpful visuals to focus on during your baby's emergence into the world.

Breathing through this stage might feel like a gradual process, but it will not necessarily take any longer than holding your breath and using strained, purple pushes to bring your baby down. Have patience with your body and your baby and know that breathing through this stage will relax the sphincters and optimise the amount of space your baby has.

Forced, strained pushing causes tension in the sphincters of the birth path which reduces the amount of space the baby has when moving down. The baby will move through the birth path as and when the next part of the birth path is ready, and the uterus will push accordingly at just the right time for this. This also gives your baby the time and space to make any adjustments to their positioning – an intuitive human instinct – imagine you want to walk through a narrow doorway. As you approach the doorway, do you maintain the same position and hurry through without rearranging how you are standing or do you slow things down and turn your body in order to fit through more comfortably and more easily?

Practise birth breathing on the toilet. Having a stool movement is something you do regularly, and your body knows how to do it. Having a baby is something you do far fewer times in your life, maybe only once, but your body knows how to do it just as perfectly as it knows how to perform every other natural function. Practising birth breathing when sitting on the toilet is also a good way to demonstrate to yourself during your pregnancy, how your natural expulsion reflex muscles do things for you with no effort on your part at all and that pushing or straining can slow down the natural intended process of many things.

Visualise the rose opening, focus on that and your cyclical breath, trust what you now know and surrender to the power of your birthing body as your uterus pushes your baby down and out.

With forced, strained pushing, a woman breathes in, holds her breath and tenses most of her body, causing the gripping and propulsion of the baby's head. Immediately after she releases the breath she was holding, the sphincters release and her baby moves back up the birth path. With birth breathing, she breathes in through her nose and the uterus pushes the baby down. The next breath in is taken through the nose, thereby avoiding any extreme tensing and releasing of the sphincters around the baby.

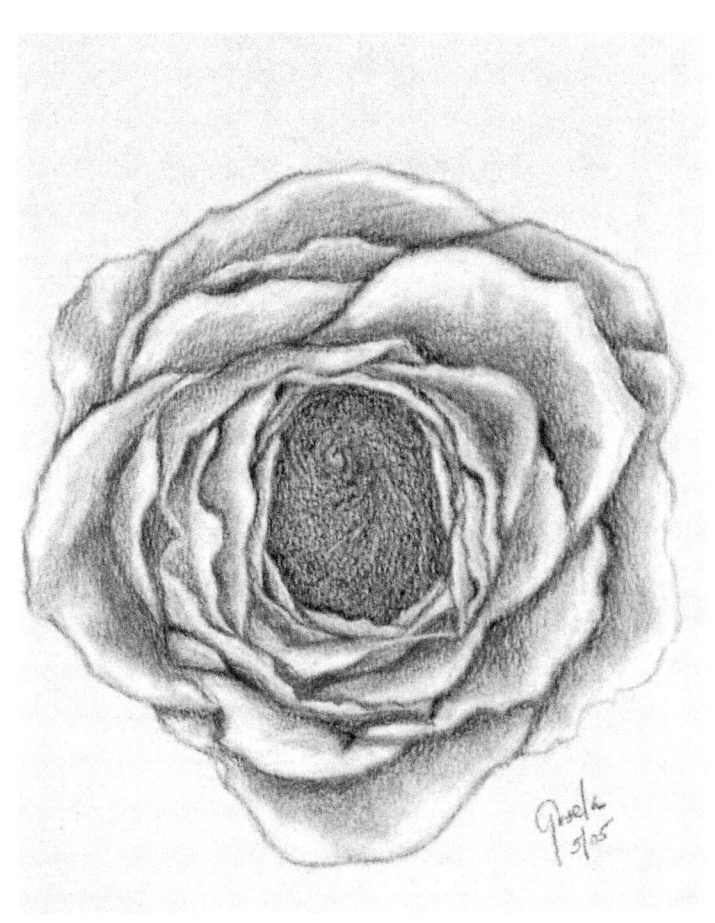

(Opening rose imagery from Hypnobirthing - The Mongan Method)

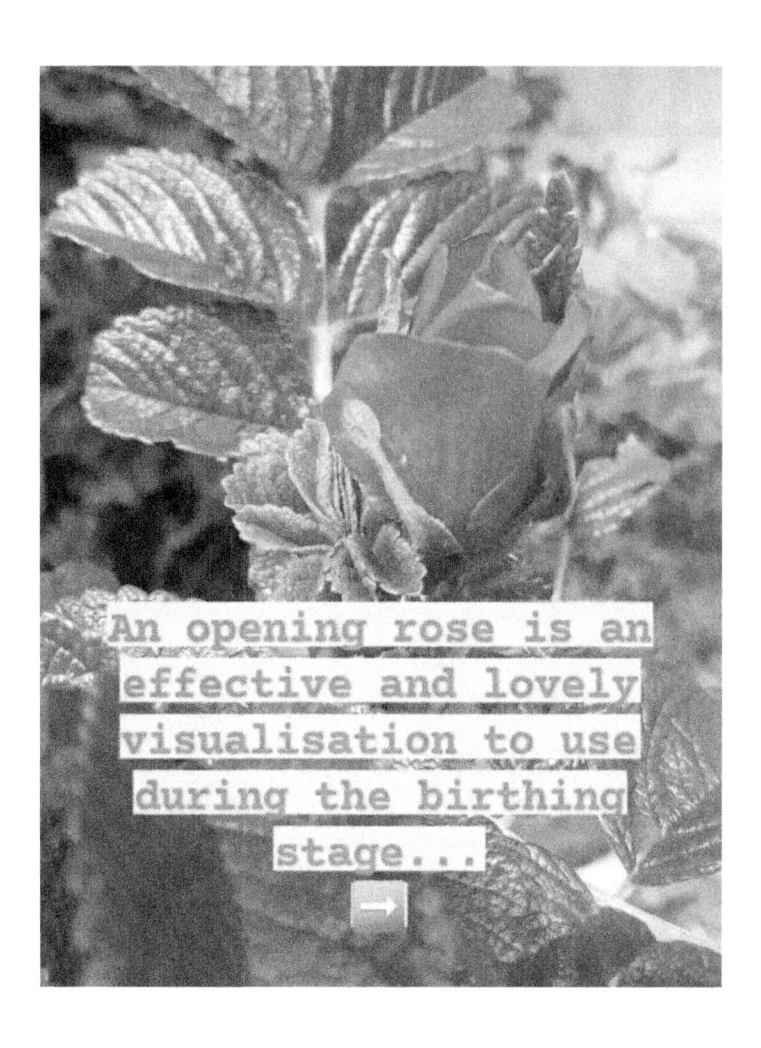

An opening rose is an effective and lovely visualisation to use during the birthing stage...

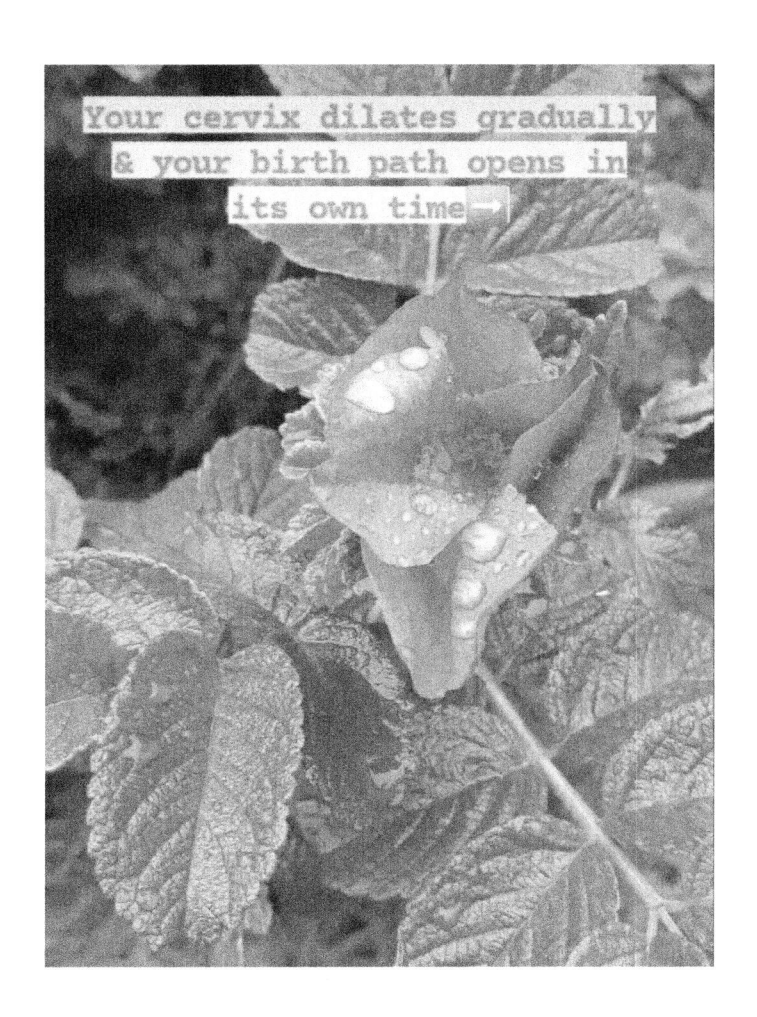

> Your cervix dilates gradually & your birth path opens in its own time →

> Give yourself permission to surrender to the power of your 🌸 body 🤍

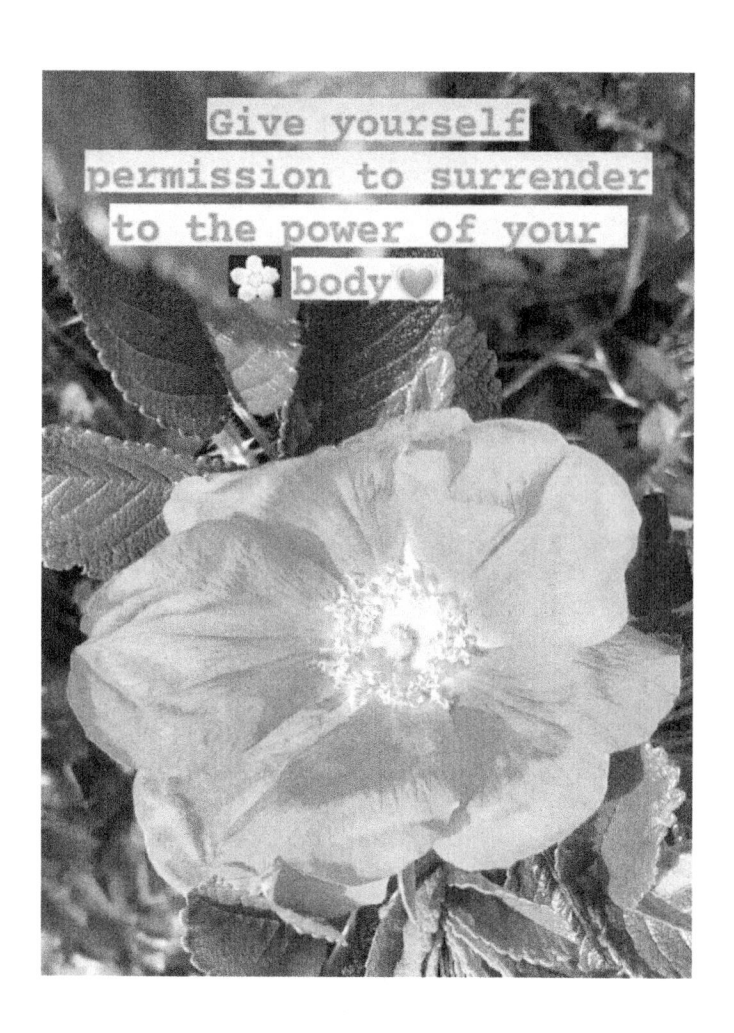

Four things I wish I'd known before giving birth.

That I might have a show - You might notice a thick, pinkish or blood-streaked discharge and this could be a sign that labour is imminent. It occurs when the mucus plug comes away from your cervix. It's called a show and it can happen several days before labour starts. Mine happened in Asda at exactly 40 weeks. Orla was born 5 days later.

The Purple Line - A vertical, purple line appears on a woman's lower back & grows longer as she dilates. See Hour 10 for more on this.

No bladder sensation - During my labour for the first time in my life, I did not feel any urge to urinate. Until someone suggested to me that the cause of the fullness and pressure I was feeling might have been because I had a full bladder, I did not consider this. I didn't feel the need to go for a wee and so I hadn't been. Empty your bladder regularly during labour even if you don't think you need to and get your partner to remind you to do this.

Baby period - Four days after my daughter's birth, we found some blood in her nappy. The health visitor assured us this was normal. Babies are exposed to their mother's oestrogen levels in the womb and once born, those hormone levels drop sometimes causing minor vaginal bleeding in baby girls. It can start any time from 2-10 days of life. This is normal and called false menses. The blood-tinged or pink discharge should not last more than 3 or 4 days

My uterus is the strongest part of me; it knows what to do and it works in harmony with nature.

HOUR 12

How do you feel about labour and birth now and how do you think it will be?

At the very end of your last hypnobirthing class, it was time to put pen to paper again – on the back of the sheet your practitioner kept since your course started. She will have handed you the sheet folded or front side down and asked you the above question again. What are your words now? Here's what other expectant parents said:

Prepared

Ready to put what we've learnt into practice now

Excited to give birth!

More relaxed

Like we have the tools we need to have the experience we want

Confident

Supported

Empowered

Knowledgeable – knowledge is power!

I feel like before we started the course, I was expecting the midwives to tell my partner what she needed to do at each stage but now it's as if we will tell the midwives how she wants things to be and what they can do to help my partner

Positive

I can do it!

Calm

I can breathe through it

Ready for change

Natural

In tune with my body

Trust

Powerful

Able

Free of fear

Peaceful

Strong

I have the toolkit that I need now

Capable

Happy

Free of tension

I feel like I can ask questions and make my own choices

Even if I need a C. section, I will know how to stay calm

My birthing body
does
everything
at exactly the
right pace
for
me and my baby.

Parents' Promise

I promise to love you – unconditionally

I promise to protect you – for your pain hurts me more than my own

I promise to guard and to guide you – materially, mentally and morally

I promise to foster soundness and strength – in your health, your head and your heart

I promise to catch you doing things right, and let you do things your way no matter how messy or asymmetrical

I promise to applaud your accomplishments – whether they be anonymous for nobody's eyes, or world famous, for the Nobel Prize

I promise to be a good example always – for there's no telling what act or attribute you might emulate

I promise to be honest, open and direct

I promise to be a pillar of courage and a pillow of comfort

I promise to explore the world with you, explain the world to you and expect the world of you

I promise to be a fortress in which you can hide, a friend in whom you can confide and a parent in whose heart you'll find love and in whose eyes you'll find pride

By David Teplow

(For Nathan, Alisha, Lily and Henry)

Ways To Practise And Prepare For Your Hypnobirth

MP3s

MUST : Subconsciously 'listen to' your 'Aurora Relaxation for Birth' MP3 once a day at bedtime as you're drifting off to sleep.

MUST : Listen to your 'Words of Conscious Re-Affirmation' MP3 during the day when you are feeling alert – for example at breakfast time or when you are getting ready for your day.

Enjoy listening to the other Rose Method MP3s as and when you like.

BREATHING TECHNIQUES

MUST: Practise your Esdaille Resting Breaths (Lavender, short breath, 3,2,1 relax) as and when needed – to be used for relaxation during pregnancy and between surges during labour and birth.

MUST: Practise at least 3 surge breaths (long breaths with equal inhalation/exhalation & balloon or waves visualisation) – to be used during your surges in labour.

MUST: Practise birth breathing when on the toilet together with the opening rose or rosehip flower imagery – to be used during the birthing stage when you can feel your body pushing your baby down.

OTHER RELAXATION TECHNIQUES / ANCHORS / DEEPENERS

Practise The Birth Companion's deepener as often as you like.

Practise your preferred Ultra Deepening Technique/s – (thermometer 40-0, hypnobirthing valve and numb hand techniques).

Practise soft soothing strokes with your partner as much as you like. From 37 weeks, if your birth partner extends their touch out to the side of your face, ears, breasts and décolletage, this can encourage labour to start and for surges to become stronger once you are already in labour, due to the combination of powerful endorphins and oxytocin being released simultaneously.

Relaxed hands technique

<u>FURTHER PREPARATION</u>

Prepare your perineum by doing perineal massage with or without an Epi-no (a few minutes per day from about 34 weeks).

From about 35 weeks, spend a little time visualising and focusing on your baby being in an optimal birth position at the front of the uterus, with their head down and their back to your belly.

BELIEVE IN YOUR BODY, MIND AND BABY'S COMBINED ABILITY TO WORK TOGETHER! YOU'VE GOT THIS!

I look forward
to meeting and
holding my baby,
their skin to
my skin.

The Rose Method Birth Stories and Testimonials

'Everyone should do this. My second birth was an amazingly enjoyable experience that I felt in control of. Despite going against all advice, I birthed my daughter in a pool in my lounge at home with absolutely no pain, with total confidence in my choices & ability to birth naturally. Worth every penny!' - Jenny, Poole

'I truly loved the experience & think everyone should do Hypnobirthing!' - Charlotte, Bournemouth

'I felt relaxed & calm throughout & we definitely feel that the classes helped us. We would recommend these classes to everyone.' - Alexis, Bournemouth

'Thank you for everything, especially showing me childbirth isn't a scary thing! **Thanks to you I was able to stay calm, in control & enjoy the experience of childbirth.'** - Aisha, Hants

'I knew what was happening & what to do. The breathing helped & surges started four minutes apart. Imagining a wave got me through every surge. I can honestly say I felt no pain.' - Maria, Bournemouth

'The midwife said I was one of the calmest people she'd ever seen.' - Gemma, Bournemouth (Gemma was my first ever client)

'Couldn't have been more different from my first experience. All my surges seemed to be over in seconds. Thank you so much.' - Susie, Christchurch, UK

'We went to the midwife-led unit as the midwives who came to the house didn't believe I was in labour. I breathed him out in the pool with just gas & air. Thanks again - such a positive experience.' - Clare, Southsea

'I'm trying to comprehend how different, positive & amazing it was. Thank you for such a wonderful gift' - Clare, Bournemouth

'Bourne Calm transformed my life. Coming from a family who feared the pain of birth, Rose opened my eyes to the truth that birthing can be calm, enjoyable and a connective loving experience. I was incredibly lucky to meditate through my entire labour, at my own pace in flow and rhythm with my body and its needs. Since, I have gone on to train as a yoga teacher and I teach a lot of the tools I learnt from Rose in my yoga classes, knowing the huge benefits of what it can do. Thanks so much, Rose for giving me the greatest gift of a beautiful calm delivery of my baby girl. x' – Jamii, Bournemouth.

'Thanks to Rose and her Hypnobirthing course, I had the birth that I had always hoped for but didn't quite believe was possible (despite all the peaceful Hypnobirthing videos I watched and stories I had read).

Rose was very flexible and our sessions were booked over several weeks. This meant I didn't have to rush there from work and that I had time to reflect and practise what I had learnt each week.

My first birth was not an experience I wanted to repeat. This birth was completely different in every way...

During early labour, I relaxed and laughed with my family, managing the surges via the breathing and visualisations I had been practising. We decided to head to The Haven once my surges *were getting quite close together and stronger. I wasn't sure it was the right time as the pain was manageable and certainly nowhere near how my first labour felt, but I (thankfully) listened to my husband.*

Originally I had not wanted to be examined, but I decided to allow an examination when I arrived at The Haven as the midwife was quite sure I was not in established labour, as I was very relaxed and laughing in between surges.

Much to her surprise, I was 4cm with a very thin cervix, so I decided to make use of the birthing pool straight away. Still feeling very relaxed and managing only with the water, breathing and visualisations.

Things then kicked up a gear and with the help of a little gas and air towards the end, our beautiful daughter was born peacefully in the birthing pool an hour and a half after arriving at The Haven.

I can honestly say that waiting for them to complete the paperwork and discharge me (nine hours later) was the most stressful part of the birth!

I thoroughly recommend you visit Rose if you are looking to have a positive birth experience.' – Candice, Bournemouth.

'I contacted Rose to do a refresher course after using hypnobirthing with my first child four years ago. I was a little fearful that because my first birth had gone so well it couldn't possibly this time! However, my second birth was so similar to the first, thanks to the techniques I learnt, and I felt much more confident about it. I managed to use the birthing pool, breathing, and gas and air for the final pushes. It really couldn't have gone better, and I owe Rose a thank you for giving me back a positive head-space regarding birth, as well as making me feel more empowered about my choices.' – Megan, Christchurch.

'Doing hypnobirthing with Rose has really changed our mindset about birth. We are so pleased we did the course with Rose. She's very informative and friendly.' – Vanessa (online course via Zoom)

My husband and I recently took part in the Pregnant Pause Retreat with Rose at Bourne Calm Hypnobirthing, and we cannot speak

highly enough about it. I knew I wanted to do a hypnobirthing course because I was so fearful of giving birth and had only heard positive things from people who had made hypnobirthing a part of their plan, no matter what birth they ended up having. Aside from all the wonderful tools we learnt from the course itself (to help keep calm and feel more in control through labour, and about birth in general) the three-night retreat helped consolidate our learning whilst having a relaxing weekend away. The other couples were lovely, and we also had plenty of time to ourselves. It was great for the dads too as they really felt so much more involved and learnt everything we did to feel confident in what to do when the time came to support us through labour - instead of panicking! We felt totally pampered, as the retreat included a massage, pedicure, and facial for the mummies-to-be, a couples' pregnancy yoga class, and amazing food provided throughout. The setting was perfect, and we were sad when it was over! Rose was a lovely, caring host and we left feeling so much more prepared and excited about the birth of our baby boy. ***I think this should be mandatory for all pregnancies!!!***
Thank you so much, Rose. x' – Amy.

'I can only thank Rose for the knowledge she passed on to me, without which my birth would not have been the amazing experience it was. Thank you Rose also for the way in which this knowledge was shared. With these things and my own practice, I managed to go through a night of contractions (surges as you'll learn they're called), visualising, with the whole process happening in the way I had already been imagining for weeks that it would, and moving my body in a way that made those sensations feel totally safe and well, and feeling like my body was simply preparing for the morning. I knew baby would come in the morning. The surges went from very spaced out (hourly, to every 15 minutes, then every five minutes, within a matter of two hours), which was a new experience to me also as my first labour had taken 24 hours.

This time, labour itself, with intense surges, lasted about one hour, and the birthing was 15 minutes with no pushing - I got a bit insecure at this stage and asked the nurse, 'Am I good? I don't have to do anything?'
And *she replied reassuringly, 'No, your body's doing the doing.'*
Then I continued to trust all that I'd learned about my body and mind. And baby arrived without blood or tearing, which was a dream for me, having my eldest to care for and play with. It felt like this was really the only way I could ever give birth again - at home and with the hypnobirthing techniques. **My partner also can't recommend it enough** *as he felt safe and secure too. His hypnobirthing soothing strokes massage on me was also so good that at one point he was moving away, and I remember saying, 'Come back.'*
Baby arrived in the sac, safe and sound, at home. Mum, baby and the whole family had an amazing experience. Rose, thank you so much! I couldn't have done this without you.' – Livia, Poole.

'Hi Rose, What an experience – my word! Mum and baby worked in perfect harmony. I wanted to thank you for providing us with such a fabulous skillset. The process was remarkable, and hypnobirthing was, without a doubt, a major factor in such a successful, calm birth. If you ever need a reference or would like me to speak with a couple or the expectant fathers to give my take on it all, I would be very happy to. It is the least I can do. The birth was special and there was not a thing I would change. It was so calm, and when things got tough, we remembered your voice and vital words to keep us on track to a wonderful conclusion.' – Ian (Livia's partner).

'The hypnobirthing course with Rose was amazing. Rose was very flexible, warm, friendly and professional. The environment where she taught was very relaxing. I now understand much more about birth and feel relaxed and confident about it. I consider the course should be a mandatory tool everyone should get before giving

birth.' – Teresa, Bournemouth.

'This is the second time I've done a hypnobirthing course with Rose. I was so pleased to hear that she was still running courses via zoom throughout the pandemic. The zoom calls were equally as beneficial as face to face, and I actually found it so much easier as I didn't have to arrange childcare for our little girl. Rose was very accommodating, and an evening zoom call was perfect. Hypnobirthing is amazing and I'd recommend it to anyone. **It completely changed my views about labour, and I've had two wonderful experiences.**' – Laura, Bournemouth

'The hypnobirthing certainly did help me as visualising the waves and hearing James read the passages out to me certainly got me through the contractions. It was amazing... Totally pain free... Totally different experience to the first.' – Hannah, Verwood

'I am over the moon with both of my experiences. No intervention was needed in the end. As you know, I was considering the sweep or balloon to induce me. I was checked over, only to be told I was already having surges and was 2 or 3 cm dilated, so I let nature take its course and this is how it went:

My cramping started at around 4 or 5am on the Saturday and the surges came and went. At their closest they were eight minutes apart. This time around, I felt the surges and used the balloon visualisation (with Amy's first birth, she didn't even feel her surges!) The surges slowed after a while Mark and I went outside and within 15 minutes, they had come back stronger and more frequent. I then told Mark we had to leave for the Haven, knowing we were getting close to meeting our baby. I put in my headphones and we drove there. When we arrived at 8.45am, I was 5cm dilated already, the bath was being run and I was busy with my breathing. Within an hour in the water, Emily's head was born *after what must have been just three or four J-breaths. However, her shoulder got stuck in my pelvis and I was rushed out of the water and onto the bed. With a bit of movement, she was freed and after about one more J-breath she was born with no pain relief nor stitches required! She is already a delightful, happy, content baby. Again, Mark and I would like to thank you for all you have done to make birthing both of our babies the most magical and worry-free experience. I will absolutely continue to be hypnobirthing's biggest advocate.' - Amy, Poole (Amy went on train as a hypnobirthing practitioner).*

'I wanted to give a guy's impression of Hypnobirthing. I truly believe it helped us to have a relatively relaxed and straightforward labour and birth. Before we did the Hypnobirthing course, Charlotte was extremely scared and doubted her ability to get through it with or without pain relief and drama. This in turn caused me to worry about things that could go wrong, and I had no idea what support I could give. We decided to give Hypnobirthing a try because we thought anything that could relax us and get us 'in the zone' would be a huge help on the day. We were a bit sceptical about the course as we honestly thought it sounded to good to be true. How wrong we were! Hypnobirthing was great in the weeks leading up to labour by helping Charlotte to relax, believe more in her own body and ability to give birth, and to sleep better in the last few weeks when it's pretty uncomfortable for a pregnant woman.

Charlotte found that listening to the birth affirmations most mornings for the last few weeks, helped to cancel out the negative voice in her, and gave her the

extra confidence she needed to not be scared when it happened. She still had some of the nerves and anxiety a lot of women naturally experience surrounding childbirth, but she was far more in control of these thoughts and emotions. Also, I was able to say some of the birth affirmations to Charlotte before and during labour. Charlotte stayed comfortably at home until she was getting contractions every four minutes. We then couldn't believe it when we got to the hospital and Charlotte was 7 or 8 cm dilated. The next seven hours saw a very determined and focused mother-to-be, who was in control, used the breathing techniques taught to get through the surges and finally bring our beautiful daughter into the world. Charlotte only had to use gas and air during labour - we were expecting to have to use every pain relief available! Dulcie was very calm and content when she was born, which I put down to the fact that Charlotte was relaxed and focused. This helped ensure it wasn't a traumatic experience for mother or baby. We had a water birth, which was truly incredible. You hear a lot of dads say that they feel like a spare part during labour. The Hypnobirthing course gave me advice on things I could do before and on the day itself. Thank you, Rose. We are truly grateful for your guidance and advice, and for helping us to understand more about labour, and techniques to get through it! We cannot believe that our beautiful daughter is finally with us. Now we just need some advice on dealing with sleepless nights!' – Rob, Poole

'Rose, Thank you for all your help with our one-to-one hypnobirthing. It was an amazing experience. The hospital staff even thanked us afterwards, for making it an amazing experience for them too. It really helped me to stay focused and we delivered our beautiful boy just the way we wanted to at Poole hospital. I used gas and air and only needed that at the very end. Three hours 58 minutes total labour and birth time. Thank you for everything xx I will be ready for round two in a few years xx.' – Simone,

Bournemouth.

'Hi Rose, I just wanted to let you know that I had a beautiful baby girl, Evie, yesterday – up in a hospital in Leeds, as we were there for the weekend. Despite the change of venue, I had a midwife-led labour with gas and air and was in hospital at 2.30pm and Evie was born at 8.50pm. I wanted to say thank you for what I learnt on your course as it definitely helped me to have an easier and more natural birth.' – Ali, Bournemouth

'Our story....

We had quite a traumatic first birth with our son and we wanted to try and approach our second birth with a positive head on, so this is when we approached Rose. I didn't know if I would be able to do all the visualisations, as I knew I was rubbish at keeping my head focused on one thing, but I realised that even if we just went into birthing feeling positive and not scared, I would have been really happy.

We knew we would be on a monitored ward because of previous complications, but through hypnobirthing and Rose's reassurance, we were able to realise that a calm birth was possible, even in a monitored environment.

We played the affirmations every night and practised the breathing and visualisation techniques and began to feel far more positive. By the fourth session with Rose, we started to look forward to the birth.

As we approached and went past our due date, we began to fear that we were heading for induction again, but after some acupuncture, reflexology and spicy food, contractions started. Although, they were really irregular, and I thought that they would stop like before, so I went to bed and just breathed through them. At 3am, they were coming every five or six minutes, and I realised this was the real thing, although they were easy to breathe through and then carry on as normal in between. I even made some food and pottered around the house for a bit, before my brother, who had stayed to look after our other little one, said he thought it was time for us to head to the hospital as the surges were four or five minutes apart!

I still believed we must be in the very early stages as they were really easy to breathe through, and I hadn't even noticed they'd got so close together. I put the affirmations and guided visualisations on my iPhone and listened to them in the car on the way there.

As we got to the unit, we told them we were hypnobirthing and they were totally supportive. We were left alone for an hour, as we looked so calm. I guess they just thought we were in the early stages too.

I had some gas and air to help through some more intense surges (I think I must have been going through transition at that point) and kept listening to the guided visualisations and affirmations on my earphones, which helped to keep me focused.

When they finally came to check us, the midwife looked up and smiled and asked if we'd had a long labour last time. I nodded and she replied that it wouldn't be this time and very soon the baby would be here. I was already 8 cm, and five minutes later I was at 10! And she was crowning!

They totally respected that we were hypnobirthing and at this point just told me to listen to my body. So, I turned to lean on the bed (as I'd seen on one of Rose's birth videos and my friend had also recommended this). My waters broke straight away then, and two breaths later, she was born - **and I really did only feel pressure then as she was born and nothing more, no pain or anything. I really couldn't believe it!**

We were so amazed that she was born so peacefully in just two and a half hours, and that I was actually able to do it!

One of the most important things that helped us was hearing other people's positive stories and seeing all the calm hypnobirths. This, in turn made us feel that it was possible for us and not a myth! So, thank you, Rose for the wonderful gift you have given us. We hope lots of other women and their partners are able to have the same experience x' – Claire, Bournemouth

'Dear Rose, **Thank you for all the skills you taught me to have a positive birth experience**. Lots of love. Xxx' – Karen, Bournemouth

'To Rose, **Thank you! You helped me achieve my VBAC!** Rose, your kindness financially enabled us to attend your course and I am eternally grateful to you. My dream came true of no second C-section, and I know a major part of that was down to the Hypnobirthing. Wishing you and your family all the best and hoping your business goes from strength to strength. You are a natural at what you do, and it worked for me. xxx' - Alice, Poole.

'I found it really helpful. I didn't need any gas and air and **felt really calm and in control.** She is such a calm, relaxed baby, possibly due to the Hypnobirthing. Thanks for your help.' – Emma, Wimborne.

'Thank you so much for playing such a big part in the birth of our daughter, Emily. I had a wonderful birth thanks to you and the hypnobirthing techniques.' – Jenny, Poole.

'Hi Rose, Hope you are well. Matt and I just wanted to let you know that on Monday 13th January at 9:20pm our beautiful baby Olivia was born. I had an amazing labour and birthing experience.

The midwives said they were amazed how calm I was and that I didn't make a noise throughout.

I went into early labour at 4am on Monday. I stayed calm and listened to your lavender script and watched some funny films. The surges were getting closer and stronger as the day went on, and by 5pm, we went into Bournemouth birth centre. I was examined and found to be 3 or 4cm dilated and confirmed to be in established labour. The surges did get intense, but I used the breathing techniques and wave visualisations to get through. I was 5cm dilated by about 8:30pm, and decided to get into the birthing pool around 8:45pm. The surges became extremely intense, so I started to use gas and air then. After just four of these intense surges and half an hour later, she was born.

Thank you so much for all of your help and advice during our hypnobirthing sessions. We feel it really did make a huge difference.' – Sophie, Bournemouth.

'Hi Rose, Our beautiful little one was born on Sunday after five hours of active labour, and I had a lovely experience! The water really helped me. ***I felt like I was in a hot tub with a glass of Prosecco, which is my happy place.*'** – Sophie, Bournemouth (second baby. Sophie's first birth story is the entry above this one).

'Hi Rose, How are you? I had my baby on Thursday!! I feel like second time around was definitely more positive and empowered thanks to Hypnobirthing. I'd been having twinges for weeks. I then had a scan which diagnosed excess amniotic fluid, so I opted for a sweep at 40 weeks. Then the next day, whilst trying to get into bed to cuddle my eldest goodnight, my waters broke. Labour came on really fast and strong with surges every seven minutes. Half an hour later, they were every three minutes. I was focusing on beathing, but at times I felt out of sync. I kept bringing myself back to my breath throughout. We got to the hospital and, 41 minutes later, he was born! Once I birthed his head, he just shot out! **Throughout the whole labour, I felt my body was doing everything automatically and it was the most surreal and amazing feeling**. I didn't get any of that with my first. Thank you for teaching me Hypnobirthing. I feel like it's helped me so much, not just in labour but in overcoming fears around the pandemic and generally helping me to relax. Thank you. xx' – Karina, Bournemouth

'My son's birth was such an incredible, empowering experience, and it's all thanks to Rose and her hypnobirthing techniques.' – Hannah, Poole.

'Rose, Just a little something to say thank you for everything! I feel like you have changed my life so much for the better. You truly care. You are amazing and an inspiration and I am so thankful that you have come into our life. Thank you so much.' – Chloë, Poole

'Just wanted to say a big "thank you" to you following the birth of our gorgeous daughter. After the four sessions of your Hypnobirthing course, my husband and I felt confident walking into the birthing suite with our arsenal of Hypnobirthing tools, and following a 30-hour, pain-relief free labour and two fantastic midwives (who by chance were both Hypnobirthing trained!)

our daughter arrived calmly and didn't cry on arrival or for the entire first week! It was a really positive experience for us all and very different to what we had imagined it would be like prior to completing the course. Thank you again.' – Ami, Bournemouth.

'They examined me for the first time, and I was ready to breathe her out. 15 minutes later, she arrived into the world. I felt really pleased that I did it all just using Hypnobirthing, my Tens machine and some gas and air, and so was able to go home six hours later. It was a complete contrast to my first birth!! Thank you for supporting me with the Hypnobirthing; it definitely made a big difference to how I approached the birth and made me feel more empowered that I could do it, even in non-ideal circumstances! Best wishes.' – Anna, Dorset.

'Hi Rose, I have to say *thank you so much for your wonderful hypnobirthing course. I had the most incredible birth journey. It was everything I could have possibly hoped for and I felt so confident, calm and empowered throughout.*
My surges started at 2am and I was able to stay in bed and rest whilst using the surge breathing.
At 6am, we called the labour line and were told Ashurst was still

closed due to midwife shortages. But I found myself unfazed and we headed to Broadlands birth centre.

The room we first went to for the initial checks was incredibly hot and I hadn't had an opportunity to eat and hadn't drunk much water, so unfortunately whilst being examined, I passed out and was sick, so I got taken to the labour ward for monitoring.

I remained calm throughout and continued my breathing and despite things slowing down in terms of my surges, thankfully after a couple of hours I was told I could return to the birthing centre and have a pool birth.

Things picked back up quickly from there and I gave birth to our little girl in the water, using gas and air for the last couple of hours. James was a brilliant support throughout, and said how amazed he was by the difference he saw in me this time around; he was very proud and also in awe.

I felt truly wonderful afterwards and was delighted to be able to return home by the evening.

I am in absolute awe of what the human body can achieve and I'm so glad to have been able to find the belief in myself to have such an incredible experience.

Our son is absolutely besotted with his new baby sister, and she is very relaxed and content.

Thank you again for helping to make this a reality for us.' - Amanda, Christchurch (course completed on Zoom during Covid-19 lockdown)

'Hello Rose,
We had a baby boy last Tuesday!
We did most of the labour at home after planning a home birth and

it was wonderful.

On Tuesday morning, we ended up popping to Ashurst to get checked out... they offered an examination (in my plan I had said none and hadn't had any from midwives visiting home so far) just to see how things were progressing so I agreed to the check.

I was at 9cm (dilated)! The midwife was so surprised, she thought maybe 3cm because I was so calm.

Anyway, we decided to just stay there to have the baby, they ran the water bath there, Joe went to get our bags, my waters broke and then I hopped in the pool and had the baby two hours later!

The second stage when I was in the pool birthing was so magical -

we had the instrumental track on repeat and Joe was by my head counting down and reminding me to breathe the baby down.

I was super in the zone and fell asleep a couple of times between surges!

I genuinely had no pain for this part apart from stinging when he crowned. No pain relief, just super calm and controlled.

The midwife said it was the calmest birth she's seen for a while

and the student had never seen a water birth before, so it was a really positive experience!

So, thank you; we definitely used so many of the techniques from the course and also just the knowledge of what was happening at each stage and also empowering us to push for the birth we wanted.'
- Jenny, Hants (course completed on Zoom during Covid-19 lockdown)

'I had two refresher sessions on Zoom with Rose when expecting our second. Loved both sessions; Rose is fun, warm, loving and absolutely brilliant at Hypnobirthing. She shared many great techniques with me. Rose even wrote a unique script just for me when something came up in the last week of my pregnancy. I thoroughly recommend Rose – she's fabulous!' – Melissa, Dorset.

'Hi Rose, I've been meaning to tell you that I woke up on Thursday morning with my waters broken and contractions every three minutes. We used the hypnobirthing techniques, and I had a bath before we went to the hospital at 9am. We took all of our LED candles and our mammoth music playlist but unfortunately, you were right, and our little one was turning around and became back-to-back. I wasn't able to hold onto my focus and after severn hours, I had an epidural (my contractions remained three minutes apart for the entire time). I ended up having an emergency c-section BUT I didn't find ANY of the experience traumatic and I thank you SO MUCH for everything that you gave us. The last part of **my pregnancy went from complete terror to absolute enjoyment once we started the hypnobirthing, and I would recommend you to everyone**.' – Joanne, Ringwood.

'Hi Rose, I just wanted to let you know that I went into labour at 8.30pm on Saturday, and didn't make a sound the whole time! **I had my eyes closed, didn't speak, and just breathed. It was SO amazing** and I couldn't recommend you enough! I had the most amazing birth experience and couldn't have asked for anything more. Please feel free to share. Thank you so much for *everything. x' - Maxine, Poole.*

'Hi Rose, Ralph arrived at 5.39 this morning after a two-hour labour. ***I thought I was going to have him in the car but made it into the pool just in time to get him out. Birth was wonderful.*** *The Haven Suite was dimly lit and I was calm and remembered all of my breathing and affirmations. Thank you for all your help.' – Rebecca, Bournemouth (course completed on Zoom during Covid-19 lockdown).*

A testimonial which shows just how beneficial Hypnobirthing is, regardless of the course your birthing takes & how much medical assistance is needed. We can't control everything BUT we can control how we react in our minds & how we feel. Well done to amazing Lisa & her beautiful baby for staying so calm throughout. Lisa & her wonderfully supportive partner Mike attended a one-to-one course with me:

'Hi Rose, I had baby Evie at 00.15 on 14th October. Unfortunately, she was born by an emergency c section under a general anaesthetic. I was in labour for 20 hours and went 14 hours with no pain relief before needing an epidural as I was not dilating. They put me on the inducing drip and made it quite strong. I was very tired so had a nap while I couldn't feel the contractions and when I woke up at 12pm, I was shaking and very unwell. They monitored the baby's head and said I had dilated to 7cm, however her heart rate had dropped too low and mine had too. I started to become very sick, so within minutes, I was being taken to the theatre. ***She is a very calm peaceful***

baby and I really believe that is all because of the hypno! It kept me so calm and in control of the pain throughout. I recommend it to every woman, especially if you are nervous or have a low pain threshold. It was upsetting that I didn't get the natural birth I had really hoped for, but using what I learnt from Rose made all the difference and kept me calm, relaxed and ready for birth. Oh also, last Tuesday night, I went to Barolo's and had the Aubergine Parmesan recipe! I talked to them about it and showed them the recipe and they sorted it for me! I will say it was delicious, and well, my waters went the next day, so I hope it works for other mums also xxx A big thank you for everything.' Lisa, Christchurch.

Another beautiful birth story - this lady was high risk due to having gestational diabetes:
'Hi Rose,
I hope you are well! I've been meaning to email you to let you know that our daughter was born last Sunday at 1pm. Thank you for all your help & advice through the hypnobirthing course. It really helped & enabled us to have such a calm, relaxed & incredible birth experience!

I never believed you when you said that people who hypnobirth have such a good experience that they would happily do it again the following week. Well now I can relate & I agree!
Right from the start of my labour, I listened to my affirmations

and music which really helped me to stay chilled & distracted. I used lavender oil as you suggested & again this helped. I was high risk and had to be monitored constantly, and the midwife was great & very respectful of the fact that I wanted to stay as mobile as possible. When we first arrived, the midwife seemed convinced that I would be going home as she thought I wasn't in established labour. However, when she examined me, she was surprised to see that I was 4cm dilated! My husband was amazing throughout the birth and found the tips you gave us useful in helping me with the visualisations and ensuring I stayed calm & relaxed. I managed to deliver with just gas and air, and the midwives were so impressed with how steady & stable baby's heart rate was throughout labour and birth, and how alert she was when she came out! Thank you so much for giving me the skills & confidence to turn something I was so petrified about into an incredible birth experience xx' - Rakhee, Bournemouth.

When things don't go to plan, Hypnobirthing helps. Here are testimonials from two of my clients for whom that was definitely the case:

'Hi Rose, I just wanted to let you know that little Jack arrived at 42 weeks and two days. Although almost everything didn't go to plan, the hypnobirthing techniques I practised were incredibly *helpful*. **At some points no one would have known I was having a surge**, because I was lying down thinking of my waves and counting in my head and reminding myself, "this is what my body needs to do." **Without Hypnobirthing I think I would have panicked** a lot more and it would have been much more painful and a longer process. So, thank you very much for the sessions. They really helped. Xxx' – Alice, Bournemouth.

'Hi Rose, Here is my hypnobirth story and pictures from the day, which I'm happy to be shared. Our birth story...
When I found out I was pregnant I watched tons of birth videos on YouTube to see what I was in for when the day arrived. Most of those were American women lying in beds, hooked up to machines with their legs pulled back by midwives and screaming while being told to push, pause and pant. This did nothing to help my anxiety over giving birth!
I heard about hypnobirthing through the hospital I was attending for my appointments and was told they do a class on the NHS and I signed up straightaway knowing little about it but feeling it would be a wise choice. The class was split into two parts and my partner Eddo and I attended the first session open minded and ready to embrace it.
After taking the first class I was immediately put at ease from the teachings of how our bodies work naturally and already I felt very calm about the birthing experience to come.
At seven months pregnant we moved house to be closer to my family. This meant that we would miss the second half of the hypnobirthing course. I searched to see if I could find anything in our new area as it turned out that the previous hospital was one of the very few that offer this course on the NHS. I kept searching and narrowed it down to a few private teachers, and was instantly drawn to Rose Hypnobirthing.
I contacted Rose, who was extremely accommodating and tailor-made a couple of sessions for us (and my mum). Rose guided us through some relaxation and breathing techniques to practise.
Throughout the remainder of my pregnancy, I listened to the hypnobirthing tracks every night and regularly practised the breathing. I listened to the affirmations and put them up around the house and my partner read me a script before going to bed (IF he hadn't already fallen asleep!) I felt extremely confident that I would have a calm and positive birth.
My due date passed, and I was patiently waiting for the first sign of labour. At 41 weeks I woke up to a small leak in my waters,

and after being checked out was advised to have an induction as there was a small amount of blood present. I really didn't want to have an induction and I felt anxious, but I felt well informed and asked lots of questions (thanks to hypnobirthing), before making a decision.

I was examined and my cervix was still far back, so I had the first stage of induction (the gel). I was advised to give it 6 hours and that the first stage doesn't always work. The midwife said I'd probably be there well into tomorrow before anything happens.

Within half an hour I was having surges every two minutes. I was in the antenatal ward amongst other women and there was no sign of being able to have the water birth that I wanted. Although I couldn't set-up our desired atmosphere with the lighting, I continued to use the Hypnobirthing breathing throughout my surges and my partner and mum supported me. At times it was off putting as there were women in the same ward screaming through their surges, but I remained calm.

My surges were coming strong and fast with barely any gap for about nine hours. Throughout this time, I was offered pain relief. I gave in to paracetamol, but it came straight back up, and I also considered some pethidine (I didn't plan on this, but my surges were so close together that I felt like I needed some rest). I didn't end up having it however, as when I was next examined, to the midwives surprise I was 4cm dilated, and was advised I could go to the delivery suite and use the pool.

During the surges I tried to relax my body and focus on the sensation. I noticed that whenever I held tension and wasn't focused, the feeling was painful however when I was focused, it was not painful, and instead felt like an intense and empowering sensation. Shortly after getting into the pool, my surges changed and I realised I needed to switch my breathing technique to the down/J breathing. I also used the visualisation of the flower opening.

I was asked to come out of the pool to give birth due to the bleed and the size of our baby. This made me anxious as I thought that I had more chance of tearing out of the pool. I was completely zoned out during this part of the birth and just surrendered and trusted that my body and baby knew what to do and that everything would be ok.

Within two hours, our beautiful baby boy emerged head first, with his hand around his face and talking before he was completely out. I had a bleed in the third stage, so I ended up having syntocinon to help the placenta out, and seven people rushed in to help, which would have likely panicked me before, but I used the breathing throughout this time to remain calm and it really helped.

Our baby boy is super calm and relaxed which I believe is due to the Hypnobirthing. **I was amazed that I had no pain relief and did not tear at all.** *(I say this as I only managed the perineal massage a few times!) Now thinking back about my birthing experience,* **I really don't think I would have coped without Hypnobirthing and putting in the practice.'** - Lucy, Bournemouth.

'Hi Rose, H made her arrival on Sunday. She was born in the birth pool at home, established labour was two hours 35 minutes with no pain relief or intervention and I didn't tear. Thanks again for the refresher – **it was just what I needed and I can't imagine having such an amazing birth if I didn't have all the knowledge from your** *course.'* - Kirsty, Poole (second-time client).

'Hi Rose, We had a baby girl. It was a totally different experience from before and hypnobirthing had a huge part in that. **Although it was a C-section, I felt so in control and was able to communicate with the midwives/doctors in between my surge breathing.** So, thank you. Although it ended up being via C-section again, I was ok with that and I was awake for it so my husband was able to be with me this time. I was naturally induced (balloon placement) and that worked really well; I dilated to 4 cm within five hours but that was as far as I dilated unfortunately, and baby's heart rate kept dropping so they performed an emergency C-section. We are both doing really well, although recovering from a C-section takes time! Thank you for your sessions. **It certainly helped me to stay calm and made me realise that having a surgical birth isn't a bad thing**; it was necessary for my baby to be born safely. xx' - Adele, Poole.

'Rose, I just wanted to say Baby R was born and he's perfect. I actually ended up on the IV drip due to the labour being quite long and waters breaking some time earlier, **but I managed the entire thing** *pain relief- and drug-free using the visualisation and breathing techniques you taught me.* Baby was actually found to be breech at a 36-week scan and we had to check the position of the placenta. I am so, so pleased I stuck to my guns and refused the forceful ECV turning procedure a number of times. Reflexology, yoga and a little swimming, plus just letting my body do what it needed to, and he turned head down on the Friday before he was born – I felt him move! I just wanted to say thank you for giving me the confidence to trust in my own body. *I think without Hypnobirthing, I would have been far more easily swayed to go immediately with what the doctors said.* xx' - Hannah, Poole.

'Hi Rose, Just to let you know that our baby girl was born at 1.50pm on Friday. *The hypnobirthing was incredible, and totally saved me during the surges and pushing.* I did use some gas and air which helped with the surge breathing and the pool and aromatherapy enabled me to relax so much. Thanks again for everything – we shall 100% tell everyone our story about how much Hypnobirthing worked for us. Tons of love. xxx' - Vicky, Verwood.

'Oh, hey, Rose! Just thought I'd let you know our little girl arrived.

I was induced due to reduced movement but the whole process was very smooth! With an established labour of one hour 45 minutes, I found the techniques you taught me really useful and helpful. I managed to have no pain relief until I was 6 or 7 cm. From then on, I had gas and air, which I'm proud of myself for as my labour was also back-to-back so very intense! We named her Luna (she was also born on a full moon)! We enjoyed the course and highly recommend it to other people who are anxious about labour and pregnancy. **My partner was able to keep my focus throughout by helping me to remember the techniques and going through the motions with me.** Thank you very much. – Steph, Ferndown.

'Rose, Just a message to introduce you to Margot, born on Valentine's Day! Thank you so much for your course, it was worth its weight in gold as my first contractions were at 1am on Wednesday, so I had a long time to practise everything during latent labour! Andrew also saved the day reminding me of birth humming at the vital moment. It was fantastic to feel so knowledgeable and for Andrew to genuinely help me every step of the way. We went into hospital at 7cm dilated and only an hour and a half before she was born. **The midwives were so impressed by how calm baby and me both were and wished all their women were the**

same. *The Haven was empty except for us, and Margot was born in the birthing pool (and even hung out in the water upside down whilst I waited for the final pushes!) I managed all of it with only a small tear with no stitches!*
Thank you very much for your help getting us there!' – Claire, Poole.

'Rose is a truly amazing Hypnobirth instructor. I completed her course and she gave me the confidence & belief that I needed to give birth to my beautiful daughter at home in complete harmony as planned. My labour was two hours in total, **I was in complete control, and it was one of the most amazing experiences of my life.** I was never scared, and at every stage of the labour, my affirmations were prominent in my thoughts. **Hypnobirthing is the way forward and recommend this course to every pregnant woman. Spread the word!'** – Katie, Bournemouth.

'Thanks to Rose's Hypnobirthing sessions, I had the most wonderful birth. I wish I had known about her when I had my first son! It was a truly amazing experience. I still use the relaxation technique to keep myself calm and in control. I must say **there are so many challenging things in this world, and I always think that** *my Hypnobirthing labour was much easier than all of them!'* – Akiko, Poole.

'Rose is a lovely, warm-hearted, chatty person. I took my partner along with me to her course; he was very sceptical at first and asked lots of questions to begin with, but he was soon converted and now recommends it. By coming along with me, he also learnt the tools and techniques needed for a smooth, controlled labour and the role he needed to play. We really enjoyed doing this together and practising the techniques. My partner was so helpful when I was bringing our baby into the world, as he also understood what was happening to me and my body (because of what we learnt on Rose's course). We had such a positive birth experience. When I first heard about Hypnobirthing, I was unsure about it, as I previously had an emergency C-section and didn't get my happy ending, so was convinced I would be going for an elective C-section this time to get my baby out safely. It's only when a friend said, "Have you heard of Hypnobirthing?" We first went along to one of Rose's taster sessions to see what it was all about. I'm so glad I did this despite a lot of family members worrying about my choice. My midwife totally let me get on with it – I did have continuous monitoring in hospital, but by using the techniques, I managed to not let this worry me or distract me. My labour flew by! Don't get me wrong – when I first went into labour, it was a shock, and it took me about an hour to get my head in the game, but once I did, there was no looking back. **I had an all-natural, back-to-back labour. One of the midwives commented on how well I looked afterwards. I beamed a** *smile and said, "Hypnobirthing!"* She probably thought, "You potty lady", as most people do. Even I did until I knew what it was all about. The name Hypnobirthing doesn't do it justice. ***If you're going to do any course, I would highly recommend this – it's worth the money, time and effort.'*** – Olivia, Ringwood.

'My wife Holly and I are currently on a Hypnobirthing course with Rose. We are learning so much and really look forward to our sessions, relaxing in the calm, tranquil summer house at Rose's. We are really excited to welcome our baby into the world using this proven formula for a natural birth. Rose's calm nature and depth of knowledge is just what we need to prepare for our baby's arrival.' – Andy, Christchurch.

'Rose has made us feel so much more confident with our birth. Thank you, Rose – I'm still practising with seven weeks until my due date. xxx' – Kelli, Christchurch.

'Rose was such a welcoming, calming and supportive teacher.
My husband and I did our course with Rose, and I really can't thank her enough. I don't think we could have got through our labour without the techniques that she taught us.
We had planned a homebirth with a pool, but unfortunately our little boy had other plans! I started at home using Rose's breathing techniques and listening to her MP3s, which couldn't have set me up any better for the events that were to happen later on in my labour. I was extremely calm and in such a positive and excited place while I was home, my midwife couldn't believe how well I was doing. Unfortunately, our little boy decided to have a poo, and the decision

was made that I needed to be blue-lighted into Poole. I surprised myself with how well I was able to cope with this, as the last thing I wanted was to go into hospital, but Rose had prepared me so well to be able to divert from my original birth plan whilst still keeping hypnobirthing going. At this point, my surges had become very intense but I still felt in control. Once at the hospital, I managed to dilate to 10 cm with no pain relief; I just used my hypnobirthing. I am surprised how I was in my own little hypnobirthing bubble; I didn't know how many people were around me; I didn't know when other complications happened; I was just listening to what my body needed to do, and was very focused. After a long labour and without going into too much detail, I ended up having to go into theatre for a C-section, which I thought would have been my worst nightmare! Don't get me wrong, I did have a little wobble at that point, but we soon got back on track with our hypnobirthing. We even took our MP3s into theatre and carried on. Our little boy arrived safely and we are all well. I want to thank Rose from the bottom off my heart because if I had not had the help from Rose, I know I would not have been able to deal with all the unplanned events during my labour and our little boy wouldn't have had the stress free labour he ended up having. Rose also really helped my husband with techniques that he used to help keep me calm and relaxed. He was amazing and was my rock the whole way through. (Rose, he didn't fall asleep at all!)

The week before my due date, I did have a little panic that I wasn't going to be able to get through the birth. We messaged Rose on the Sunday evening, asking if we could have a top up session and she managed to fit us in the next morning which I was so thankful for. I felt so much better afterwards, and I then went into labour less than 48hours later! Thank you again, Rose. We really appreciate all your help and Barnaby can't wait to meet the amazing lady who helped his mummy and daddy xx' – Holly, Christchurch

'Hi Rose, Just thought I would update you! I got my hypnobirth! Our baby girl was born on Thursday afternoon, in water at home as planned! She weighed 7lb 5oz, which is good for 37 weeks! And

she is gorgeous! It was all lovely & quick. Thank you so much! x' – Emma, Wimborne.

'Hiya Rose, Well, what a few days! I gave birth on the 9th at 8.13pm. She weighed 7lb9. Labour started at about 4 am. I just had gas & air & 45 mins of pushing. It just took over me. It was amazing! So, thank you for all your help & support xxx' – Gemma, Bournemouth.

'I just wanted to say thank you so much to Rose and to hypnobirthing. I can't recommend this enough. I have just given birth to my perfect baby boy and the birth was beautiful. It was everything I had hoped for and more. I was relaxed and felt in control. My husband was a crucial part of the birth and talked me through our relaxation techniques in between the surges. Hypnobirthing taught him helpful things to say - to the point that the midwife actually said she'd been just about to say something when Nick said something even better and she'd think, why didn't I think of that? So, she just left us to it! My labour was two and a half hours long, which I'm told is pretty quick for a first-time mum! And I had the water birth I was so hoping for. I am so grateful to Rose and to hypnobirthing for giving my son such a lovely welcome to the world. Thank you so much, from mother, father and son xxx' – Jenny, Bournemouth.

'Rose is an excellent practitioner! I had a really calm birth that took just under two hours with no pain relief until the end and then just a little gas and air. It was a very different experience from my first birth! **I feel that this course caused the key difference in my mindset and how in control I felt throughout.** xxx' - Miranda, Bournemouth

'Our baby was born yesterday at 2.49pm. I managed to stay at home for almost all of it and used the pool and all the Hypnobirthing techniques. I received lots of compliments about my breathing. When I reached 10 cm dilated, my waters broke naturally. Then they took me to hospital as the last stage was really quite long, and I didn't have the 'pushing' sensation. It turns out she was back-to-back , and so two midwives, my mum and my partner helped to guide me to 'push' her out naturally - it took 45 minutes. They had so much faith in me. It was the most surreal, challenging and beautiful moment of my life when she came out. Thank you so much for giving us the tools to use Hypnobirthing & having a natural birth. The body is amazing! And it sure does know what to do! xxxx' - Jemma, Brighton

'I wanted to send you a big thank you for all the relaxation & breathing techniques that you taught me.
'All of a sudden, I knew what was happening & what to do.
The breathing helped & my contractions started at three minutes apart.
At the hospital, I was told I would be admitted as I was 4cm dilated. Imagining a wave washing over me as I breathed in & rolling out as I breathed out, got me through every contraction & I can honestly say I felt NO pain.
When my partner came running down the corridor, I wept in relief & then my waters broke. My baby had been waiting for his daddy.
Once my waters broke, I was given gas & air which helped my breathing & concentration. No other pain relief was used. It just wasn't needed!
Eventually, I felt my body pushing the baby out all by itself. I used birth humming to help. I was then transferred, (to central delivery from the midwife led area of the same maternity unit), because after two hours of pushing, my heart rate went up. I pushed my baby out naturally 10 minutes later - he was perfect.
The breathing techniques have been used for so much more since the birth itself.

- The birth humming helped for the first no.2 post birth.
- The surge breathing helps all the time when baby is crying but was particularly helpful in the first few days of breastfeeding.'
Thank you for your wonderful course & everything you taught me. xxx' - Maria, Bournemouth.

Review from one of my clients who was induced and successfully continued to use her Hypnobirthing techniques and stay in her Hypnobirthing mindset:

'Hi Rose,
Our homebirth didn't happen, but I wanted to tell you how helpful the Hypnobirthing was regardless.
My blood pressure had been getting higher, so I was sent in for a check at the hospital the day before the estimated due date. I hadn't realised my waters had been leaking for two days as it was a small amount. When I went in for the check-up, they kept me in to be induced.
The hospital felt horrible and clinical and so far away from the lovely fairy lights and pool set up we had at home.
Once in the birthing room, we made it as homely as we could. We turned all the lights down and had our lavender room spray and battery fairy lights with us.
They started the drip at 7am and broke my waters. I was hooked up to a monitor and drip for the whole labour & birth, but I kept mobile and on the birth ball.
I managed with just the Hypnobirthing breathing and TENS machine. The contractions were strong from the drip being turned up quite high, because they were in a rush to get me going as I had been leaking waters for more than 24 hours.
I put on a playlist that I'd made which was a mix of Hypnobirthing tracks & other very calm music (which I'd also been listening to at home every time I did my Hypnobirthing breathing practice or had a candle-lit bath). I can't explain the difference having this on made! I was suddenly much calmer and in control - it made me feel more relaxed like I had been at home. I got into my zone & then

started using the gas and air with the breathing I was doing. This was at 3.30pm.

At 5pm, I told the midwife I had to push. She looked at me like I was mad and said, 'no' and for me to get back on the bed because I was still only 4cm. They had estimated that my cervix would dilate by half a centimetre per hour with the drip.

I got off the bed then anyway & told her again because at that point my baby's head was coming out!

He was born then, and I managed it with the Hypnobirthing breathing and the gas and air.
I was so pleased and proud!
Even though it wasn't the homebirth we wanted, we were so much more in control and avoided many interventions.
My partner has also found it a massive help. He was so informed and able to make decisions that he would have had no idea about otherwise.
Thank you for all your help and guidance in helping us to bring our little boy into the world.'
- Rose, Bournemouth.

'I had an amazing experience. My baby was born at home & delivered by her father. Couldn't have planned it better.' – Sam, Bournemouth

All reviews and testimonials have been shared with permission.

Let others know what you thought of the book

Now that you've read it, it would mean a lot to me, if you'd share your honest opinion about my book here:

Amazon: www.amazon.co.uk

Find my book and scroll down to the reviews' section.   Thank you.

This book is available in paperback, ebook and audiobook.

Find Rose online

Here are Rose's online links:

www.bournecalm.com
rose@bournecalm.com
www.facebook.com/rosehypno
www.linkedin.com/in/bournecalm
www.instagram.com/bournecalm_the_rose_method
www.x.com/bournecalmhypno
www.tiktok.com/@bournecalmbirth

ABOUT THE AUTHOR

Rose Byrne

Rose has been passionate about positive antenatal preparation since 2007. Pregnant & scared, she stumbled across a birth story that would change her life forever. Two years later, learning that there was still no one in her area sharing the empowering antenatal course that had led to her calm birth experience, Rose made it her mission to bring hypnobirthing to East Dorset.

With 14 years' experience as a hypnotherapist & an award-winning antenatal educator, Rose is one of the UK's longest-running hypnobirth coaches. As well as preparing expectant parents for calm birth since 2010, she also trains & mentors others to teach The Rose Method.

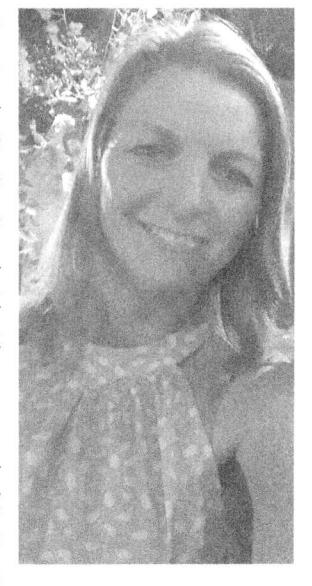

This is her first book. It's available in paperback, ebook & audiobook.

Printed in Great Britain
by Amazon